The Scientific way to managing obesity

The Scientific way to managing obesity

Dr. Mini Sheth
(PhD)

Ms. Nirali Shah
(BSc, PGDHMI, ADSE)

A Sterling Paperbacks

STERLING PAPERBACKS
An imprint of
Sterling Publishers (P) Ltd.
A-59, Okhla Industrial Area, Phase-II,
New Delhi-110020.
Tel: 26387070, 26386209; Fax: 91-11-26383788
E-mail: sterlingpublishers@airtelbroadband.in
ghai@nde.vsnl.net.in
www.sterlingpublishers.com

The Scientific Way to Managing Obesity
© 2006, *Mini Sheth*
ISBN 81-207-3189-1

All rights are reserved.
No part of this publication may be reproduced, stored in a retrieval system or transmitted, in any form or by any means, mechanical, photocopying, recording or otherwise, without prior written permission of the authors.

Printed and Published by Sterling Publishers Pvt. Ltd.,
New Delhi-110020.

Foreword

There is growing concern for the rapidly increasing number of overweight and obese people world over. This is because the condition is positively correlated with a number of disorders which may result in a shorter life span or may affect the quality of life in the long run. In order to be a healthy and useful citizen, it is essential to acquire knowledge regarding the problem of obesity, its monitoring, assessment and management which is the corner stone for tackling the entire issue.

As more and more studies confirm the importance of proper nutrition in the management of obesity and associated disorders, the need arises for a current, accessible reference in this area. This book is an excellent example of efforts to present the available relevant current literature on obesity and its management for nutritional professionals, dieticians, physicians, medical and nursing students.

In its nine chapters, the book presents a clear and systematic account of current concepts of obesity, its dietary management and issues related to eating disorders arising out of it. These chapters elaborate on the current theories and etiological aspects of obesity, measurement of obesity, its complications and the preventive and management aspects of obesity. The book also gives additional information on eating disorders, obstacles in weight loss, fad diets and myths.

Salient features of this book include wide ranging discussion on the problems related to obesity and approaches to handle them in the light of the current scenario. It is rich with a lot of basic information that can be used as a ready reckoner for all interested in therapeutic nutrition.

At the end, the book also presents a large number of sample menu with modifications in common food preparations.

With all these features there is no doubt that this publication would be an extremely useful reference material for students of nutrition, dietetics and paramedical courses. The book may also attract the attention of the common public as the content is of general interest.

I compliment the authors for their unstinted efforts in bringing out this book that contains a wealth of useful information in a brief and concise manner.

Professor Pallavi Mehta
Department of Foods and Nutrition
Faculty of Home Science
The M S University of Baroda, Vadodara.

Preface

This book is written out of concern for all those who care for good health especially for those who desire to maintain a normal body weight and wish to lose weight. Obesity is a complex health problem and unless it is understood well, its management may not always lead to its success.

There is no doubt that overweight / obesity is positively correlated with a number of health related disorders and one needs to maintain normal body weight if a disease free life is desired.

Having a physically fit body is certainly not an issue that is based on impulses and it does not happen to anyone by chance. A conscious and persistent effort on the part of the individual to maintain a normal body weight through appropriate knowledge of health foods, their amounts and a regular exercise programme are the hallmarks of a healthy life.

Why is adherence to a weight loss diet extremely difficult for some and not so difficult for others? The chapters on causes of obesity, its theories and types will answer such questions and throw light on the mechanism of appetite control.

Selection of appropriate tool to measure obesity is also an important component of a good weight loss programme. A wide variety of techniques have been elaborately discussed in this book.

Body weight reduction has been a challenge for all those who desire to lose weight either from a health point of view or from a cosmetic point of view. One can see a mad rush at the so called weight loss clinics that promise for a rapid weight loss. Individuals enrolled at such clinics do succeed initially only to return to their initial body weights. Such individuals also try out other unhealthy methods of weight loss that lead them into various types of eating disorders and health related problems. The book has also elaborated on the various eating disorders commonly experienced in all age groups.

An individual approach to management of obesity seems to be the keyword in achieving success. A cooperative client and a determined dietician will successfully reach the targeted goal.

Dr. Mini Sheth
Ms. Nirali Shah

Acknowledgement

I am thankful to the Lord Almighty for giving me the energy and patience to write this book. Thanks are due to Dr. Pallavi Mehta, a senior professor in the Department of Foods and Nutrition for writing the foreword for this book. Her constant guidance and encouragement is worth appreciating. I am grateful to Prof. U.V.Mani, Head, Department of Foods and Nutrition for his encouragement and support.

My sincere thanks are extended to Dr. Vikas Dosi and Dr. Rupal Dosi for sharing their views and resource material for writing this book.

I thank the young and enthusiastic dietician and co-author of this book for her lasting support until the completion of the book.

I would also like to acknowledge the patience and love extended to me by my husband Kiran and sons Shashin and Shalin while the manuscript was being written.

I sincerely acknowledge Sterling Publishers for their willingness to publish this book for the welfare of the student and general population.

The co-author offers her *vandana* to *Laxminarayan Deva* for divine intervention and blessings during writing.

I respectfully thank my teacher and principal author Dr. Mini Sheth for providing me with the opportunity to work on this book. My mother, Harsha and my father Dr. Hiten Shah, a successful author of several technical books, had constantly encouraged me to complete this book. I take this opportunity to sincerely thank them.

Dr. Mini Sheth
Ms. Nirali Shah

Contents

Foreword   *v*
Preface   *vii*
Acknowledgemnent   *ix*

1. **Introduction** -------------------------------- 1
2. **Types of Obesity** -------------------------------- 9
   1. Android and Gynoid Obesity
   2. Developmental and Reactive Obesity
   3. Juvenile Onset Obesity and Adult Onset Obesity
   4. Lymphatic Body Type
3. **Theories and Etiology on Obesity** -------------------------------- 13
   1. Regulation of Appetite
   2. Theories of Body Weight Regulation

   Etiology of Obesity
   1. Heredity and Genetic Factors
   2. Biological Factors
   3. Physiological Factors
   4. Psychological Factors
   5. Social, Cultural and Economical Factors
   6. Other Factors
4. **Measurement of Obesity** -------------------------------- 30
   1. Body Weight
   2. Body Mass Index (BMI)
   3. Waist to Hip Ratio
   4. Measurement of Body Fat
   5. Ponderal Index
   6. Broca's Index

7. Corpulence Index
8. Lean Body Mass
9. Body Density Measurement
10. Saggital Diameter

5. **Complications of Obesity** ----------------------------- 45
    1. Heart Disease and Stroke
    2. Diabetes Mellitus
    3. Hypertension
    4. Hypercholestrolemia
    5. Gall Bladder Disease (Cholelithiasis)
    6. Dyslipidemia
    7. Certain Types of Cancers
    8. Sleep Apnea and Other Respiratory Problems
    9. Osteoarthritis
    10. Emotional Disturbances and Social Stigmatisation
    11. Reduced Fertility and Pregnancy Complications
    12. Restricted Mobility
    13. Mechanical Disability
    14. Gallstones
    15. Fatty Liver
    16. Skin Disorders
    17. Other Co-morbidities

6. **Management of Obesity** ----------------------------- 55
    Strategies for Management of Obesity
    1. Assessment of Excess Weight
    2. Willingness and Commitment by the Subject to Reduce Weight
    3. Estimation of Energy Requirement
    4. Setting Realistic Goals for Weight Loss
    5. Behaviour and Motivation Therapy
    6. Dietary Modifications
    7. Careful Exercise Plan
    8. Compliance on the Part of the Subject
    9. Record the Progress
    10. Deviation Analysis in Case of Weight Loss Failure and Counselling for the Deviations

Other Methods Less Commonly Employed
   1. Psycho Therapy
   2. Drug Therapy
   3. Surgery
   4. Gastric Balloons and Jaw Wiring

7. **Eating Disorders and Obstacles** ----------------------------- 85
   1. Eating Disorders
   2. Anorexia Nervosa
   3. Bulimia Nervosa
   4. Binge-eating Disorder
   5. Compulsive Overeating
   6. Night-eating Syndrome
   7. Nocturnal Sleep Related Eating Disorder
   8. Pica

   Obstacles in Losing Weight
   1. Weight Loss Plateau
   2. Depression and Stress
   3. Prevent Hypoglycemia and Trigger Foods
   4. Lack of Exercise
   5. Weight Cycling

8. **Fad Diets and Myths** ---------------------------------- 102
   Fad Diets
   1. The Atkins Diet
   2. The Hollywood Diet
   3. Grape Fruit Diet
   4. Cabbage Soup Diet
   5. A Three-Day Diet
   6. Fruits and Vegetables Diet
   7. Myths and Realities

9. **Approaches to Healthy Diet** ----------------------------- 108
   1. Protein Rich Recipes
   2. Low Sugar Sweets
   3. Low Fat Recipes
   4. High Fibre Cuisine
   5. Iron Rich Foods
   6. Low Calorie Foods [Approx. 100 Kcal]
   7. High Calcium Food

Appendices	128
Appendix 1.	*128*
A. Standard Weight and Height Tables	128
B. Mean Height-Weight Tables for Well-To-Do Children and Adults	129
C. (i) Standard Weight (kg) for Men at Various Heights and Ages	130
(ii) Standard Weight (kg) for Women at Various Heights and Ages	
D. Recommended Dietary Allowances	131
E. Food Pyramid for Good Health	132
F. Food Items Containing Energy	133
G. Food Items Containing Proteins	134
H. Food Items Containing Crude Fibres	135
I. Food Items Containing Fat	136
J. Potassium (K) Rich Foods	137
K. Sodium (Na) Rich Foods	138
L. Iron Rich Food	139
M. Calcium Content Food	140
N. Comprehensive Food Exchange List	141
O. Milk Exchange	141
P. Vegetable Exchange	142
Q. Vegetable B Exchange	142
R. Fruit Exchange	143
S. Cereal Exchange	144
T. Meat and Pulse Exchange	144
U. Fat Exchange	146
V. Miscellaneous - Per 100 gm. edible portion	146
Appendix 2. Standard Measurements	*147*
Appendix 3. Common Terminologies and Phrases Associated with Obesity	*148*
Appendix 4. Tips and Suggestions	*154*
References	156

1
Introduction

Obesity is a chronic condition that arises out of excess accumulation of body fat and in most cases giving rise to chronic degenerative diseases such as diabetes mellitus, hyperlipidemia, cardiovascular problems, kidney and liver diseases, osteoarthritis, and urinary stress incontinence. Certain types of cancers also have its etiology in obesity.

In addition to health factors, other potential consequences include psychological problems such as low self-esteem, social withdrawal, depression and eating disorders. Statistics show that obesity is assuming epidemic proportions globally, both in developed and developing countries, amongst adults as well as children [Table 1(a,b), 2 & 3]. Unlike the western countries especially USA and England where there is tremendous increase in the prevalence of obesity in the past decade (25-30%), in India and other Asian countries the prevalence though on rise is low comparatively. The prevalence of childhood obesity in India ranges from 3.9% in New Delhi to 8.4% in Meerut (Figure 1a) whereas in adults the prevalence of obesity ranges from a low of 3.9% in Haryana to 17% in Mysore women (Figure 1b). This data is however not collected at one point using uniform methods. The origin of obesity lies in the family lifestyle factors imposed on us by technological advancements. In the developing countries like Asia, the problem of obesity is multifactorial. It is associated with increasing urbanisation, with dramatic changes in the trends of dietary consumption patterns and lifestyles, particularly in terms of reduced physical activity.

Most working women are unable to meet the demands of the family and tend to purchase the ready-to-eat foods available over the counters. Frequent consumption of ready-to-eat meals with high calorie content result in "Fat Families". Although the causes of obesity may vary from genetics to lifestyle factors, it ultimately results from excess energy intake as against energy output.

It is believed that intake of 200 kcal daily beyond the normal requirement for the said individual can result in weight gain of 15 kg in 2 years. Weight gain is a very gradual process and if no brakes are put, one can become morbidly obese and its reverse is certainly not an easy task.

Physiologically, obesity in adults is a consequence of increase in the size of the adipocytes whereas in children there is a 2-4 fold increase in the number of adipocytes.

Sustainable management of obesity should be a long term process based on correct diagnosis of the causes of obesity in an individual, although a firm determination and cooperation on the part of the subject remains the hallmark of the treatment.

Sprawling weight-reducing clinics all over the urban cities that promise a rapid weight reduction fail to satisfy many clients in the long run as most of these programmes do not include a balanced low calorie diet. Often they aim at rapid weight reduction that does not have a strong base in the principles of weight loss management. The individual, though may lose weight rapidly, sustainability is rarely seen. Depending upon the individual case history, a management strategy needs to be worked out that may comprise drug therapy, surgery, behaviour modification along with nutrition education programme.

In order to prevent the population from becoming morbidly obese, the government and private institutions should take immediate steps to create awareness in the population. A regular health check-up programme should be organised and educational programme should be conducted for eating health foods. Mandatory nutritional labelling may also help the subjects choosing the right kinds of foods to suit their calorie needs.

In many institutions where food is catered to the employees, supervision by dietician for healthy food preparation and serving should be encouraged.

Scientists are documenting the global "fat" problem from China to Australia to Egypt to remote islands of the Pacific and beyond. In 1995, there were an estimated 200 million obese adults and 22 million obese children worldwide. By 2000, the number had skyrocketed to more than 300 million. In developing countries, it is now estimated that more than 115 million people suffer from obesity-related problems, including type 2 diabetes, heart disease and obesity-related cancers. According to the National Institutes of Health, in the US alone, child obesity has increased by more than 1 per cent per year over the past decade with an estimated $99.2 billion in future health care costs. "We're looking at a ticking time bomb of chronic disease," said LaVelle, noting that a recent World Health Organization study found that obesity is now estimated to have increased 50 per cent over the past seven to ten years.

The prevalence of overweight and obesity generally increases with advancing age, then starts to decline among people over 60. This is because of either the onset of certain chronic disease or due to insufficient intake of food due to the problems of mastication, less mobility to buy foods and reduced physiological functions due to advancing age.

Various theories have been postulated for obesity to have its basis. The next chapter will highlight most of them.

Table 1a: Prevalence of Overweight and Obese in Asian and Other Countries.

Country	Group		Prevalence		Reference
	Age Group	Number Studied	Overweight	Obese	
Korea		720	10-20 %	20%	25
Malaysia	9-11 years	84	22% boys at risk 16.3 % girls at risk	—	13
Iran	Adult Diabetics	85	8%	3%	67
	Adults	15005	Men – 42.6% Women – 38.1%	Men – 14.4% Women – 29.5%	32
Dhaka	2-10 years	5000	—	7.6%	
Sri lanka	Adults			Men – 3.8% Women– 6%	16
China	Women 1999 Adults			Women-11.6% Increased from <10% to 15% in just 3 years	16 22 (Int)
Pakistan	Adults			Men - 13% Women – 23%	16
Japan	1974-93			Increased from 5% to 9.10 %	16
Thailand	1991-93			Increased from 12.7 to 15.6%	16

Table Contd...

Table 1a Contd...

Country	Group		Prevalence		Reference
	Age Group	Number Studied	Overweight	Obese	
England	1980-95	Men		Increased from 6% to 15.3 %	17
		Women		Increased from 8% to 17.5 %	
USA	1976/80 – 88/91	Men		Increased from 24.1 to 31.7%	17
		Women			
	Adult		64.5%	30.5%	
	Men		67.2%	27.5%	3 (Int)
	Women		61.9%	33.4%	
				Increased from 13.3% to 30.9%	3 (Int)
	1960-2000 20-74 years		Increased from 31.5% to 33.6%	Severe obesity increased from 2.9% to 4.7%	
	Children (6-11 years)		15.3%		
	Adolescent (12-19 years)	15.5%			

	Number Studied	Over Weight	Obese	Reference
South Asia	Women		3%	14 (B)
Sub Saharan Africa	Women		13%	14 (B)
Latin America and Caribbean	Women		35%	14 (B)
Central Eastern Europe and the Commonwealth of Independent States	Women		42%	14 (B)

Table 1b: Prevalence of Overweight and Obese in India

City	Group		Prevalence		Reference
	Age Group	Number Studied	Overweight	Obese	
Bangalore	Coronary Artery Bypass Graft (CABG) Patients	100	———	6%	43
New Delhi	7-9 years	1238	8.24%	6.22%	33
	15-45 years	>2500	25%	9%	40
	14-17 years	4300	26%	3.9%	48
	7-12 years	664	———	7.8 %	23
Meerut	Adults	1152	28%	8%	22
	10-19	1500	———	8.4%	
Punjab	15-45 years	>2500	21%	9%	40
Haryana	15-45 years	>2500	12%	3.9%	40
Dharwad	12-17 years	1000	4.3%	6.7%	36
Mysore	Women				42
	Executives		22%	———	
	Non Executives	46%	17%		
Ludhiana	7-9 years	60	46.6%	53.3%	24
South Indian States	1975-76			Men – 2.3 Women – 3.4	16
	1988-90			Men – 2.6 Women – 4.1	
	1996-97			Men - 3.8 Women – 6	
Chennai	1981 – 98 Adolescent girls		Increased from 9.62% to 9.67%	Increased from 5.94% to 6.23%	18

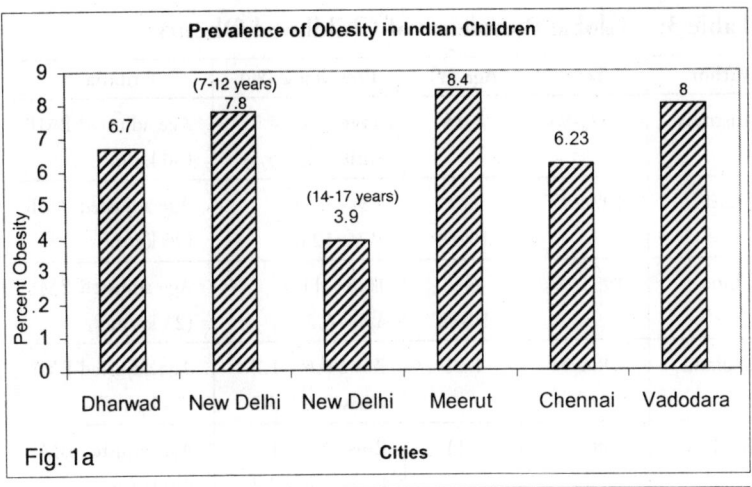

Fig. 1a

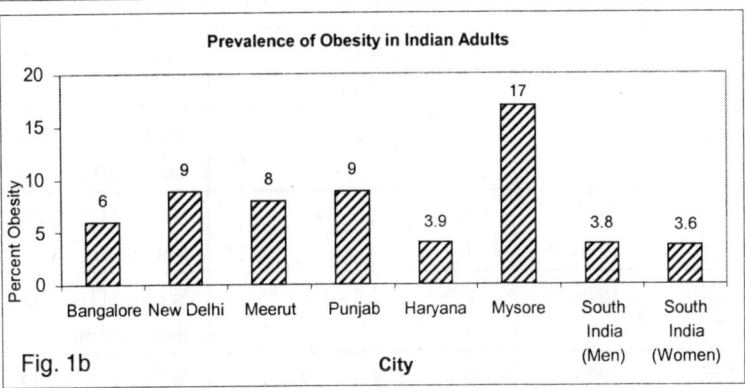

Fig. 1b

Table 2: Percentage of Overweight Females Across the World

Country	Year	Age (Yrs)	Overweight (%)
Cuba	1982-84	20-24	13.6
Puerto Rica	1982-84	20-24	23.6
Native Americans	1987	18+	40.3
Cherokee Indians	1982	18+	59.1
Pima Indians	1981-88	20-54	81
American Indians	1987	18-24	25.2
Chinese	1978-86	18+	12.8

Sources: Najjar MF and Kuczmarski RJ, 1989
Broussard et al 1995
Klatsky AL and Armstrong MA 1991

Table 3: Global Prevalence of Childhood Obesity

Author	Year	Age (Y)	Prevalence (%)	Criteria
Australia	1985-95	7-15	Boys: 1.4 – 4.7 Girls: 1.2 – 5.5	Age adjusted BMI (30 kg/m^2)
Brazil	1974-97	6-9 10-18	4.9 – 17.4 3.7 – 12.6	Age adjusted BMI (25 kg/m^2)
China	1991-97	6-9 10-18	10.5 – 11.3 4.5 – 6.2	Age adjusted BMI (25 kg/m^2)
England	1984-94	4-11	Boys: 0.6 – 1.7 Girls: 1.8 – 3.2	Age adjusted BMI (30 kg/m^2)
Scotland	1984-94	4-11	Boys: 9 – 2.1 Girls: 1.8 – 3.2	Age adjusted BMI (30 kg/m^2)
USA	1971-74 1974-99	6-11 12-19	4-13 6-14	BMI > 95th % tile
Chile	1985-95	0-6	4.6 – 7.2	Wt-for-HT > 2SD from median
Costa Rica	1982 1996	0-6 1-7	2.3 – 6.2	Wt-for-HT > 2SD from median
Egypt	1978-96	0-5	2.2 – 8.6	Wt-for-HT > 2SD from median
Ghana	1988-94	0-3	0.5 – 1.9	Wt-for-HT > 2SD from median
Haiti	1978-95	0-5	0.8 – 2.8	Wt-for-HT > 2SD from median
Morocco	1987-92	0-5	2.5 – 6.8	Wt-for-HT > 2SD from median
Japan	1970-96	10	Boys: <4 – 10 Girls: 4 – 9	>120 % of std wt.

2
Types of Obesity

Classification of obesity helps in making meaningful comparisons of weight status within and between populations. It is useful for identifying the groups or individual with increased risk of mortality or morbidity. It also helps in developing appropriate management strategies and evaluating the interventions.

Obesity may be classified as under:
1. Android and gynoid obesity
2. Developmental and reactive obesity
3. Juvenile onset and adult onset obesity
4. Lymphatic body type

1. Android and Gynoid Obesity

This classification is based on the distribution of body fat, which may have a genetic origin.

Android Body Type

The obesity in which the fat is accumulated in upper part of the body is known as android obesity, sometimes it is referred to as upper body obesity or apple shaped obesity. This type is frequently observed in most men and only a few women.

The characteristics of android body type include broad shoulders, strong muscular arms and legs, a narrow pelvis and narrow hips. Waistline does not curve inwards so the trunk has a somewhat straight up and down appearance. The android persons are usually energetic and are able to work for long hours and such people have anabolic metabolism, that results in fat accumulation in the upper part of the body. Such males have increased production of male hormones.

Android obesity can be assessed by using the anthropometric variable such as the waist-hip ratio. Other sophisticated techniques such as MRI (Magnetic Resonance Imaging) and CT Scan (Computed Tomography) can distinguish between the intra-abdominal fat from the subcutaneous fat. A positive correlation exists between the waist circumference and the visceral fat. Simultaneous increase in waist and hip measurements means the ratio is stable over a period of time inspite of considerable accumulation of visceral adipose tissue. Thus, waist circumference provides crude index of absolute amount of abdominal adipose tissue whereas the waist-hip ratio provides index of relative accumulation of abdominal fat. A high degree of accumulation of abdominal adipose tissue especially visceral adipose tissue is associated with glucose intolerance and hyperinsulinemia resulting from insulin resistance.

Results of a study of middle-aged men indicated that a large number of metabolic abnormalities were found in visceral obese men and were associated with substantial increase in the risk of coronary heart disease. The atherogenic metabolic risk markers included fasting hyperinsulinemia, increase apolipoprotein B concentration and increased low density lipoprotein. These factors were associated with a 20-fold increase in the risk of developing coronary heart disease in initially asymptomatic middle-aged men followed over a period of five years.

Gynoid Body Type

The obesity in which the fat is accumulated in the lower part of the body is known as gynoid obesity, sometimes referred to as lower body obesity or pear-shaped obesity. Gynoid obesity is generally seen in females.

The characteristics of this body type are small to medium shoulders, a narrow tapering waistline and wide hips. Weight gain tends to occur on thighs and buttocks which leads to pear shape.

There is more of estrogen in such body type, with a relative deficiency of progesterone hormone. This leads to fat deposition and cellulite around the hips, thighs and buttocks.

Gynoid women tend to crave food that are high in fat and refined sugars which further helps in weight gain.

It is now well established that a high proportion of abdominal fat (especially visceral fat) is a major risk factor for coronary heart disease, type 2 diabetes and related mortality. Whereas accumulation of body fat in the gluteofemoral region commonly found in premenopausal women (with gynoid obesity) is not a major threat to cardiovascular health.

2. Developmental and Reactive Obesity

Developmental obesity starts in early childhood and continues in the adult years. As the child grows older more and more fat gets deposited in various parts of the body. Such children grow more tall and look older than their age.

Reactive obesity is attained if the child has undergone any disease or is suffering from any of the emotional disturbances. However, during this period the body weight undergoes fluctuations and does not remain stable.

3. Juvenile Onset Obesity and Adult Onset Obesity

Juvenile Onset Obesity
It is observed that children who are overweight are more likely to become overweight adults. In juvenile onset obesity there is increase in size as well as number of fat cells. It begins in the last three months of fetal life, continues in the first 3 years of life and at adolescence.

Adult Onset Obesity
Adult onset obesity results from hypertrophy of fat cells alone. The greater the number of fat cells greater the hunger. A pharmacology intervention coupled with other management strategies will work better in treating such cases.

4. Lymphatic Body Type
The characteristics of such body type is that the limbs have thick puffy appearance and the bone structure is not visible. It seems that there is a large proportion of fat deposited in the limbs that is responsible for such an appearance. Such body type persons have gained their weight since childhood. There is an inefficient lymphatic system that causes fluid retention and such individuals appear more fat than they really are.

Such persons have craving for dairy fat products which overload their lymphatic system and cause gain in weight.

3
Theories and Etiology on Obesity

1. Regulation of Appetite

The appetite of an individual is normally controlled by two centres of hypothalamus namely the feeding centre and the satiety centre. When there are hunger sensations in the body, the individual initiates feeding in response to the detection of hunger. The eating behaviour continues until there is a signal to terminate the meal. Hence, satiety is attained.

After a subsequent inter-meal interval, the endogenous fuel is depleted and the sensations occur again.

The food intake in human beings involves different factors. This initiation and termination of feeding is affected by the signals sent to central nervous system. The brain serves as the organiser and integrator i.e. balancing the output and input of the nutrients. The hypothalamus plays an important role in the regulation of macro nutrients. The neurotransmitters like serotonin, epinephrine, norepinephrine, influence food selection. Knocking out gene for dopamine B-hydroxylase which is necessary for the production of epinephrine and norepinephrine has shown to bring about a change in the regulation of appetite leading to increased food intake.

Some peptides that are released during or after meal have been implicated in providing signals for satiation and satiety for specific nutrients.

1. Neuropeptide Y: When injected into hypothalamus increases the food intake and inhibitors of this 36 amino acid polypeptide decreases the food intake.
2. Polypeptide Orexin A and Orexin B are known to increase food intake
3. Melanin concentrating hormone, a 19 amino acid polypeptide is also known for increasing the food intake.
4. POMC (Pro Opiomelanocortin) derivative and CART (Coccain Amphitamine Regulated Transcript) both decrease the food intake.
5. CRH, the brain hormone that stimulates ACTH also inhibits food intake.

Although serotonin is known for bringing about satiation, knocking out of its receptor $5HT_{2C}$ brings about an increase in hunger and an increased food intake.

A research has shown the involvement of many more polypeptides that play a role in energy intake and energy output. However, their mechanism in appetite control is still not understood.

2. Theories of Body Weight Regulation

Obesity arises in a person when the size or the number of fat cells increases in the body. A normal person has got between 30 and 35 billion fat cells. When a person tries to lose fat, then it is possible to reduce the size of the fat cells rather than the number of fat cells. Hence with initial increase in the number of fat cells weight loss becomes difficult. There are various theories that explain the regulation of body weight. Some of them are explained below:

1. Set point theory
2. Enzyme and hormone theories
3. Fat cell theory

4. Lipostatic theory
5. Gut peptide theory
6. Push and pull theory
7. Theory of thermogenesis

Set Point Theory

According to this theory every individual has an ideal biological weight which the person is genetically predisposed to. Once this weight is reached, a set of signals are passed in the body to maintain the weight. It means a set point is reached. When the weight of the person exceeds this set point then the hypothalamus recognises the need to lose weight and vice versa.

The food intake is regulated in such a way that it maintains weight according to a given set point. It is generally not regulated on a meal-to-meal basis. When animals are made obese by force feeding and then permitted to eat as per their desire, their food intake is decreased until their weight is reduced to normal. Consequently if animals were starved and then allowed to eat as much as they wished, their food intake increased until their lost weight was gained. Similarly during the recovery from illness food intake is increased in a catch-up fashion until lost weight is regained. Even during fasting, body tries to conserve energy by reducing the metabolic rate to a certain extent.

The set point for body weight also seems to play a role in the overall weight gain and its maintenance. Even if the hypothalamus is injured the body weight does not increase indiscriminately and it seems that after the excess food intake the body weight reaches a plateau and the appetite mechanism operates to maintain the new higher weight.

Enzyme and Hormone Theories

When there is hyperinsulinemia, then lipogenesis takes place, which leads to conversion of glucose into triglycerides (fat).

The resulting high serum triglycerides are stored in fat cells i.e. in the adipose tissue and make these fat cells distended. This defect has been described as syndrome "X" (Sandra Cabot). According to her, "syndrome X is the chemical imbalance that makes you fat. Syndrome X is the most powerful medical reason why people cannot lose weight. Indeed syndrome X makes it virtually impossible to lose weight unless it is specifically treated".

The typical biochemical change that takes place in a person include insulin resistance, high levels of insulin in blood, abnormalities in blood lipids, blood glucose abnormalities, high serum levels of uric acid, high blood pressure and fat deposition in the abdominal areas.

When these fat cells absorb more of TG they emit a biochemical into blood stream called leptin. Leptin reduces the amount of a neural polypeptide called NPY produced in the hypothalamus. The weight of the body depends upon the ratio of leptin emitted by the fat cells, and NPY produced in the hypothalamus.

When there is too much of NPY then the lipogenesis is stimulated and TG are stored in fat cells. When there is too much of leptin, the fat storage is inhibited and energy expenditure increases.

In obesity both these levels remains elevated. However, the leptin receptors in the hypothalamus are desensitised. So the hypothalamus continues the TG storage in adipose cells and at the same time liberates NPY that continues to maintain a reflex of hunger beyond need and ultimately results in weight gain.

An increase in lipoprotein lipase enzyme is known to deposit fat into fat cells and has a probable role in raising the appetite. This holds true for individuals who are trying to lose weight thus making the process of weight loss more difficult.

Leptin, the fat hormone
The hormone leptin is made by a specific gene found in fat cells. Leptin influences the appetite centres of the brain and reduces the urge to eat. It decreases the content of neuro peptide Y(NPY)mRNA and increases the content of proionimelanocortin (POMC)mRNA in the arcuate nucleus of hypothalamus. In one family, where two of the children were massively obese their serum leptin levels were found to be very low. The genetic defect in this family was similar to that seen in ob/ob mice with a stop codon at position 133 of leptin gene. A family with homozygous mutation in the human leptin receptor gene has also been characterised by early onset of morbid obesity, lack of pubertal development and impaired secretion of both growth hormone and thyrotropin.

There is some evidence that leptin may have a role in obesity related hypertension. Transgenic skinny mice that over expressed leptin have relatively higher blood pressures when compared to transgenic litter mice. In addition, one study noted a positive correlation between the serum concentrations of leptin and blood pressure levels among patients with essential hypertension.

Leptin also seems to control how the body manages its body fat stores. Leptin signals the brain about the quantity of stored fat. Since leptin is produced by fat, leptin levels tend to be higher in obese people than in people of normal weight. One study reported that leptin levels in obese people were up to four times greater. There seems to be a diurnal rhythm of serum leptin concentrations, the values being 20-40% higher in the middle of the night than daytime. The peak shifts parallels with shifts in the timings of the meals. The levels are higher in women than in men and they decrease with age in both women and men. Serum leptin levels increase during childhood with highest concentration in children who gain most weight. Higher serum leptin concentrations are also associated with early onset of puberty. The issue being researched at the moment is why obese people are obese, considering they have higher than usual levels of an appetite-reducing hormone. One theory is that obese people are not as sensitive to the effects of leptin and may be overproducing the hormone in an attempt to compensate. Research is focusing on why leptin messages are not getting through to the brain.

Leptin production is also known to be influenced by the dietary intake. Overeating increases serum leptin concentration by nearly 40 percent within 12 hours. Fasting reduces serum leptin concentrations by 60-70 percent in 48 hours in both normal and overweight subjects. Leptin replacement therapy seems to be effective in patients with lipodystrophy and leptin deficiency. Although the anti-obesity effects in leptin-deficient rodents is explained through various studies, its role in the pathogenesis or treatment of obesity in humans is unclear.

Leptin and Diabetes Mellitus: The serum leptin concentration were similar in normal subjects and patients with type2 diabetes mellitus of the same weight.

Fat Cell Theory

The number of fat cells in an adult body is normally determined during the critical periods of growth such as the last 3 months of foetal development, in the first 3 years of life and during adolescence. After attaining the adulthood, the number is fixed and the cells thereafter can grow in size indefinitely.

Juvenile obesity is caused by an increase in the number of fat cells while adult onset obesity is caused by increase in the size of fat cells.

Obesity results when the size or number of fat cells in a person's body increases beyond and above average levels. A healthy person has somewhere around 25 billion fat cells.

When a person starts losing weight, the cells decrease in size but the number of fat cells generally stays the same. This is in part the reason that once a significant amount of weight gain takes place, it is more difficult to lose all of it. There is no returning to 'normal' because you have altered your body's chemistry. However, studies imply that fat cells can be destroyed as a result of maintaining a proper body weight for a prolonged period of time. That means you will lose weight, but it takes time to tighten up.

Lipostatic Theory

According to this theory, fat tissues signal the brain when they are satiated. When the glucose levels decrease to a certain level brain interprets this action and the need for food and hunger sensation is created. People with more fat cells eat more before they experience satiety. This mechanism involves long term regulation.

Gut Peptide Theory

This explains that the presence of food in the gastrointestinal tract releases one or more polypeptide which has an effect on the hypothalamus to reduce the food intake.

Push and Pull Theory

In the push theory, the person is knowingly and voluntarily pushing the excess of the nutrients in the body. This is just a behavioural disorder and can be treated by diet and behavioural change.

In the pull theory, there are inborn metabolic predispositions which generate false homeostatic signals leading to behaviour which makes excess deposition of fat. This overeating is due to certain metabolic factors and not because of any voluntary actions. The treatment for such disorders is complex and requires more than one approach of management.

Theory of Thermogenesis

1. BMR is one of the major outlets of energy expenditure and can vary with individual with different genetic constituents. It also varies during overfeeding. BMR increases when there is a change in ambient temperature. It decreases when food intake is restricted. Such an adaptor of the body to changing circumstances is termed as *adaptive thermogenesis*.
2. An another mechanism of regulation of energy expenditure occurs due to an opposing biochemical simultaneous reaction where formation and breakdown of the same molecule occurs, resulting in an equilibrium state of energy balance. For example the excess glucose intake is first stored in the form of glycogen in the muscles and liver. The same is used up as fuel for various activities and hence does not go in for lipogenesis.
3. The amount of brown tissue present in an individual also determines the regulation of energy expenditure as these tissues are known to generate more energy in the form of heat in circumstances such as overfeeding or changes in ambient temperature.

A disturbance in the normal regulation of appetite due to a damage either in the feeding centres or the satiety centres of the hypothalamus results in condition like hyperphagia or anorexia. In hyperphagia excessive eating occurs due to the damage to the satiety centres of the hypothalamus and anorexia results from damage to the feeding centres of the hypothalamus. (Figure 3.1)

ETIOLOGY OF OBESITY

The factors responsible for obesity are complex and varied. Hence obesity is also termed as a multifactorial disorder.

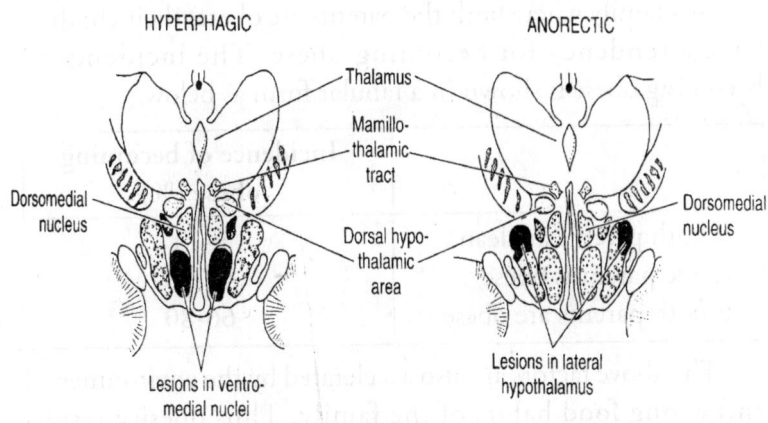

Figure 3.1: Effects of hypothalamic lesions on appetite.

Obesity can be developed at any age from childhood to adult and in either sex.

The various etiological factors resulting in obesity are as follows:

1. Heredity and genetic factors.
2. Biological factors.
3. Physiological factors.
4. Psychological factors.
5. Social and cultural factors.
6. Others.

These factors are described below in detail.

1. Heredity and Genetic Factors

These factors are the most important determinant of obesity. They influence a person's chance of becoming an obese due to inheritance of some abnormal genes. These genes cause increase in the hunger and hence there is a tendency to eat more food.

In a family where both the parents are obese, their children have a tendency for becoming obese. The incidence of becoming obese is shown in a tabular form as below:

	Incidence of becoming obese (%)
If both parents are lean	9-14
If one parent is obese	41-50
If both parents are obese	66-80

The above factors are also accelerated by the environmental and wrong food habits of the family. Thus obesity results because of the interaction between individual genetic substrate, in particular with susceptibility genes and the environmental factors. The environmental factors help the genetic factor by creating a platform to make the person obese. These genes will store the fat when there is more availability of food and the expenditure is less resulting in obesity i.e. both these factors interact and produce a trigger for the response to cause obesity.

Another factor governed by heredity is the *assimilation capacity* of persons to convert the food energy of the body into fat, which varies from person to person.

However, only 10% of obesity prevalence is because of defective genes. Today there is growing interest in searching the genes or gene polymorphism that lead to obesity. In recent years developments have occurred in identification of novel neuropeptides and other factors involved in control of appetite such as CART (Cocaine and amphetamine-regulated transcript), the orexins and the cannabinoids.

Hormones and Obesity

The hormones secreted by endocrine glands that are directly or indirectly related to fat metabolism and obesity include leptin, estrogen, insulin and the growth hormone.

These hormones function as chemical messengers which bring about the various changes in appetite regulation, lipogenesis, lipolysis, etc.

To help the body to cope up with different events and stresses the endocrine system works with the nervous system and the immune system.

Leptin
Leptin is a recently identified hormone, made by a specific gene found in the fat cells (white adipose tissue which is now recognised as endocrine gland), which controls the appetite centres of the brain and reduces the urge to eat. Although the levels of leptin are usually higher in the obese persons as they have more fat cells than the normal weight persons. Therefore in normal people an increase in leptin content reduces the food intake and increases the energy expenditure and therefore the weight is maintained. If there is a defect in the functioning of the leptin the brain does not receive signals from leptin to stop eating thus disturbing the regulation of appetite.

In some obese people although the leptin levels are higher than the normal weight people due to more fat cells, the leptin does not control the hunger and the person continues to eat and gain more weight.

When a person goes on a very low calorie diet or crash dieting then studies have shown that their leptin levels decreases which leads to increase and with the concomitant metabolic rate is reduced. Hence, when they return to their normal diet they usually regain their lost weight faster.

Other Protein Signals
Besides leptin, the other factors that may have a role in appetite control include the hormone adiponectin, resisting (which are implicated in insulin resistance), clinical7 cytokines such as K-6, TNF(ALFA) and proteins involved in vascular homeostatis (plas7minogen activator, inhibitor 1 and tissue factor).

Growth Hormone

This hormone is produced by the pituitary gland in the brain. It is responsible for individual's height and thus contributes to bone and muscle binding. It has been reported that in obese persons the levels of growth hormones are lower.

Cushing's Syndrome

The another name for this syndrome is hypercortisolism. It is a collection of the hormonal disorders that results in elevated levels of cortisol hormone. This hormone regulates many functions of the body including stress management.

The hypothalamus, which is the part of the brain sends CRH hormone to pituitary gland which then produces another hormone called ACTH. The ACTH then stimulates the adrenal gland to produce cortisol. The blood levels of cortisol are maintained by the hypothalamus and the pituitary gland. They adjust the release of the hormone as the need be. This is how the normal balance of cortisol is maintained.

Sometimes this balance is disturbed, i.e. the level of cortisol is increased which results in cushing's syndrome and can lead to increase in weight, especially in the abdominal part of the body.

Hypothyroidism

In this condition, there is not enough thyroid hormone (thyroxine) to control normal rates of metabolism. Hence the metabolism slows down. It can lead to fatigue and weakness of muscles, reducing the activity of the person. This underactivity of the thyroid gland can lead to increase in body weight.

Hypothyroidism is commonly observed in the middle age group and premenopausal women. The reduced activity of thyroid gland can be brought to normal through drugs, by modifying the lifestyle and dietary factors.

2. Biological Factors

It is reported by Dietz, 1994 that the prenatal period of adiposity rebound and adolescence appear to represent three critical period for development of obesity. The in-utero nutritional exposure has a role to play in the appetite regulation and the number of adipocytes entrained in the foetus. Late in-utero exposure to undernutrition may reduce adipocyte replication whereas late in-utero over nutrition may cause adipocyte hyperplasia. Therefore early under nutrition may affect the regulation of food intake and predispose to later obesity.

Whitake and Dietz (1998) stated that maternal obesity increases transfer of nutrients across the placenta inducing permanent changes in appetite, neuro endocrine functioning and energy metabolism in the foetus.

It is also known that infants born to diabetic mothers are fatter at birth than the infants of non-diabetic mothers.

3. Physiological Factors

There are certain critical periods during the growth and development of the person that demands increased energy intake e.g. third trimester pregnancy and lactation, during childhood, and adolescence. A person consumes more energy during such critical periods. However after this critical period passes the energy intake should actually come back to normal. If this does not happen and the diet pattern (increased calorie intake) continues over a long period of time the person gradually gains more weight and becomes obese.

4. Psychological Factors

Various psychological and behavioural problems can cause people to eat more and gain more weight. Eating may also take place when the people are stressed, bored or angry and under depression.

People having high economic status and more leisure time have a tendency to pass their time by nibbling between the meals resulting in increased weight. Frequent availability of highly palatable foods of individual choice also leads to overeating.

The obese persons have strong desire to eat much of the foods kept on the dining table but will not take small effort to move if some food is kept away which leads to increase in their weight.

Stress

Inability to recognise or express emotions such as hunger, fear, anxiety, frustrations and rejection leads to abnormal eating pattern. Stress releases increase epinephrine, which increases the amount of energy needed to overcome stress situation by stimulating large amounts of glucose, fatty acid and amino acids. If stressed individuals do not metabolise these nutrients they get converted into fat. Stress results in decreased levels of blood glucose, which leads to increased appetite and overeating as soon as the situation is over.

A person with insomnia tends to eat during night when he is awakened which leads to excess intake of food and weight gain on a long run.

5. Social, Cultural and Economical Factors

People who come from high socioeconomic group have a good purchasing power and a capacity to buy variety of foods. They frequently take expensive high calorie foods (such as ice creams, cold drinks, sweet meats, milk products, dry fruits, etc.) to express their status and gradually gain weight leading to obesity. Such individuals generally indulge in minimal physical activity.

6. Other Factors

The other factors resulting into obesity are as follows:

(a) Age

The metabolic rate of a person slows down after the age of 30 and requires less calories to maintain the ideal body weight. With the progressing age, if no change in the calorie intake as well as activity is made, the individual gains weight

Even if the body weight increases the metabolic rate does not get affected as this weight is due to increase in body fat.

(b) Gender

As males have more resting metabolic rate because of increased muscle mass than females, they require more energy than females to maintain their body weight. An average man uses about 20% more energy than females. Due to this fact men face less difficulty in losing weight than women.

(c) Eating Habits

The eating habits of certain people can lead them to obesity e.g.:

- A housewife who prepares delicious foods in kitchen and does not want the left over to be thrown may become obese. She may also nibble between meals and gain more calories.
- Some people have a habit of eating very fast and spend less time for chewing the food and in the process they consume much more food before their satiety signals are received.
- Habit of eating sweets after meals daily can also lead to gain in weight.

(d) Lifestyle Factor

When the lifestyle of the person changes from a busy life to a steady life, the energy output is reduced, however due to constant habits of earlier food intake his intake does not reduce. This creates positive energy balance. Thus men and women have a greater tendency to increase weight after the age of 50.

Due to technological revolution where everything is available at the click of the button people walk less even for the small tasks. For e.g. availability of the intercom facility at the table top prevents a person to walk to the next room.

Most business meetings take place along with major meals of the day. These meals are usually calorie densed and regular intake of such meals can lead individuals into a positive energy balance.

The availability of gadgets and machines at home, modern transportation etc. contribute to reduced energy expenditure. Besides this the type of occupation such as that of a teacher, executives etc. also lead to sedentary lifestyle. These groups of people usually have paid help at home to do the manual tasks, thus reducing the energy expenditure.

(e) Quality of Food and Frequency of Meals

The amount of food intake and its quality play an important role in etiology of obesity.

The quantity of the diet consumed may be less but calorie density of such foods may be more e.g. fried foods such as chips, *samosas*; cakes, *gulab jamum*, etc. Frequent intake of such foods results not only in a positive energy balance but may expose the individual to deficiency disorders of the vital nutrients. Ludwing et. al. (1999 & 2000) reported that high glycemic index foods like breads, cakes, biscuits, ready-to-eat cereals and soft drinks induced a sequence of hormonal events that stimulated hunger and caused overeating in adolescents.

Association between fast food consumption and total energy intake and body weight in adolescents and adults is well established. McNutt et. al. (1997) reported higher prevalence of obesity among girls (9-10 years) eating fast foods four times or more a week than those who did not due to consumption of 185-260 calories more per day.

Fast food typically incorporates all of the potentially adverse dietary factors, including saturated and trans fat, high glycemic index, high density and large portion size of foods.

The frequency of the meal is also a very important factor. A person who takes two heavy meals tends to be more obese than a person who eats four light meals.

(f) Lack of Exercises
Regular exercises play an important role in reducing the risk for obesity. Lack of exercise along with a high calorie diet can result in decreased energy output and on a long run result into obesity.

(g) Lack of Knowledge
People are either unaware about the calorie values of the food items or wrongly informed regarding the nutritive value of various foods. They have incorrect information on the energy required for various activities/exercise. Such individuals consume wrong foods, which leads them into a positive energy balance.

(h) Smoking Cessation
Smoking is believed to reduce body weight. Nicotine raises basal metabolic rate, i.e. raising the rate at which the body burns calories. However when they cease to smoke, their weight increases rapidly as they tend to curb the urge of smoking by excessive food intake.

(i) Time Availability
Due to the increased competitions of the contemporary world at various fronts of life people side track physical activity which is most essential for healthy life in order to meet the deadlines. Such commitments that are essential often does not allow the individual to spare time for routine exercises. This leads to the consumption of high calorie fast foods.

Thus, the etiology of obesity is multifaceted and its magnitude requires an appropriate management.

4
Measurement of Obesity

Obesity can be measured in many ways. The most common ways are:
1. Body weight
2. Body mass index (BMI)
3. Waist to hip ratio
4. Measurement of body fat
5. Ponderal index
6. Broca's index
7. Corpulence index
8. Lean body mass
9. Body density measurement
10. Saggital diameter

1. Body Weight

The measurement of body weight is the simplest way to assess obesity. The obesity is measured by using the weight of a person and comparing it with the desirable weight as discussed earlier in Chapter 1. If this weight is more than 20% of the desirable weight, the individual can be considered as obese.

To estimate standard weight for height: The quick way to estimate standard weight for height is to use the **Hamwi method** which provides a fairly good estimate of appropriate weight for height. The Hamwi method can be applied to adults five feet tall or taller and is calculated as follows:

For a woman with an average height of 5 feet should weigh 45 kg. And then 2.27 kg is added for each additional inch of height. Therefore the standard weight is ±10% of 45 kg.

For e.g. the standard weight for a woman 5 feet 7 inches tall would be 45 kg + 16.3 = 61.3 kg. Thus the range of standard weight for height for a woman 5 feet 7 inches tall is 55 (-10%) to 67 kg (+10%).

For a man of 5 feet the weight should equal 48.2 kg, and then add 2.7 kg for each additional inch of height. The standard weight is ±10% of this. Calculating as above, the range of standard weight for a man 5 feet 7 inches tall is 60.5 kg to 74 kg.

2. Body Mass Index (BMI)

It is also known as *Quetlet Index*. Body Mass Index is defined as the ratio of weight in kg divided to the square of height in metres.

$$BMI = \text{Weight of the person (kg)} / [\text{height of the person (m)}]^2$$

Based on the international association for the study of obesity (IASO) 2000, WHO has recommended a cut off of 23 kg/m² for Asians to define overweight. This was done due to a substantial increase in health risk found across the Asian countries.

BMI	Grades	Risk for co-morbidities
<19	Undernourished	—
19-23	Normal	—
23-24.9	Overweight	#
25-29.9	Obese	##
>30	Severe obesity	###

Source: *International Obesity Task Force (IOTF). The Asia Pacific Perspective: Redefining Obesity and its Treatment, Australia, Health Communications Australia Pvt. Ltd., 2000, p 18.*

Overweight

The BMI ranges from 23-24.9. People in this grade lead a normal healthy life and have normal life expectancy. The increase in weight does not affect their health greatly and do not generally require professional help for weight reduction.

Obesity

The BMI ranges from 25-29.9. People in this grade appear to be in good health but have less tolerance to exercise. The increase in weight can result in undue fatigue and decrease in the capacity of circulatory and respiratory system. They have problem in breathing on exertion. They can be treated by getting advice from doctors and dieticians. They have a risk of diabetes, atherosclerosis, hypertension, fatty liver, gall bladder disease, osteoarthritis etc.

Severe Obesity

The BMI is greater than 30. It is considered to be severe and a pathetic condition. Their risk for developing co-morbidities is higher than the obese. They also have serious psychological disturbances. The mode of treatment for such individuals can be pharmacological along with diet modification. However in case of BMI greater than 40 surgery may be the mode of the treatment.

Measurement of Obesity • 33

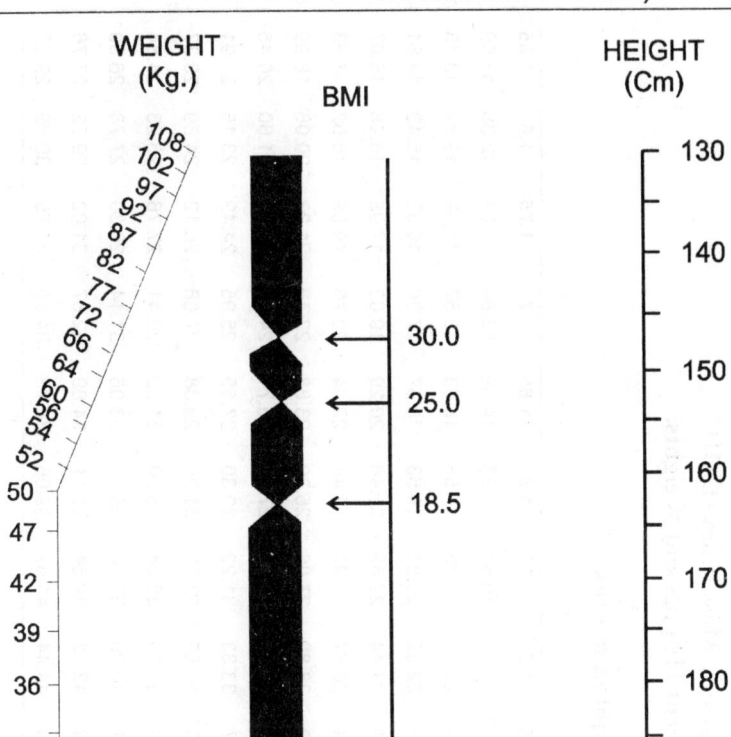

NOMOGRAM DEPICTING SAFE LIMITS OF BODY WEIGHT FOR HEIGHT
Place a ruler on the height and weight scale so that the straight edge touches the desired height and weight value.

BMI	Category
BMI<18.5	Undernourished
18.5-25	Normal
26-30	Overweight
>30	Obese

According to the revised cut off points for BMI for the Indians, the following BMI chart can be used as a ready reckoner to determine the BMI.

Chart Showing Body Mass Index (BMI) Values for Different Heights and Weights.

Height in metres

Wt.(Kg)	1.20	1.25	1.3	1.35	1.4	1.45	1.5	1.55	1.6	1.65	1.7	1.75	1.8	1.85
40	27.78	25.60	23.67	21.95	20.41	19.02	17.78	16.65	15.63	14.69	13.84	13.06	12.35	11.69
45	31.25	28.80	26.63	24.69	22.96	21.40	20.00	18.73	17.58	16.53	15.57	14.69	13.89	13.15
50	34.72	32.00	29.59	27.43	25.51	23.78	22.22	20.81	19.53	18.37	17.30	16.33	15.43	14.61
55	38.19	35.20	32.54	30.18	28.06	26.16	24.44	22.89	21.48	20.20	19.03	17.96	16.98	16.07
60	41.67	38.40	35.50	32.92	30.61	28.54	26.67	24.97	23.44	22.04	20.76	19.59	18.52	17.53
65	45.14	41.60	38.46	35.67	33.16	30.92	28.89	27.06	25.39	23.88	22.49	21.22	20.06	18.99
70	48.61	44.80	41.42	38.41	35.71	33.29	31.11	29.14	27.34	25.71	24.22	22.86	21.60	20.45
75	52.08	48.00	44.38	41.15	38.27	35.67	33.33	31.22	29.30	27.55	25.95	24.49	23.15	21.91
80	55.56	51.20	47.34	43.90	40.82	38.05	35.56	33.30	31.25	29.38	27.68	26.12	24.69	23.37
85	59.03	54.40	50.30	46.64	43.37	40.43	37.78	35.38	33.20	31.22	29.41	27.76	26.23	24.84
90	62.50	57.60	53.25	49.38	45.92	42.81	40.00	37.46	35.16	33.06	31.14	29.39	27.78	26.30
95	65.97	60.80	56.21	52.13	48.47	45.18	42.22	39.54	37.11	34.89	32.87	31.02	29.32	27.76
100	69.44	64.00	59.17	54.87	51.02	47.56	44.44	41.62	39.06	36.73	34.60	32.65	30.86	29.22

The Dietary Guidelines for Indians (1998) of National Institute of Nutrition have suggested an average BMI of a population between 21 or 22 and while that between 25 and 30 is considered overweight. The following nomogram can be used to determine the BMI of an individual by placing the ruler on the height and weight scale so that the straight edge touches the desired height and weight value.

3. Waist to Hip Ratio

This is another way of measuring obesity. The waist to hip ratio for males should be less than 0.9 and that for a female should be less than 0.85. The waist to hip ratio greater than one for both males and females is a risk for cardiovascular diseases.

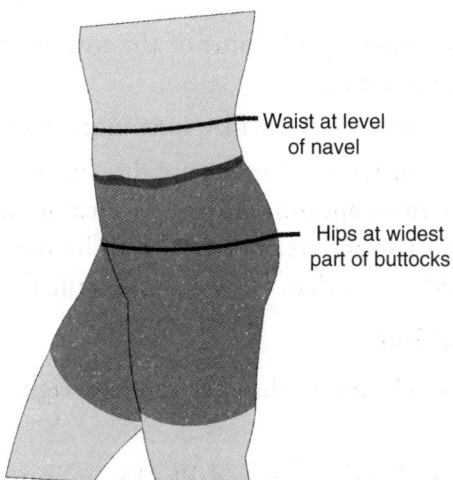

4. Measurement of Body Fat

Certain amount of fat in the body is essential for stored energy, heat insulation, shock absorption and other functions. Mostly women have more amount of body fat stored in the body than men. If the fat in the body increases more than 25 percent in men and 30 percent of the total body weight in women then they are considered to be obese. Measuring the exact amount of fat in the body is not an easy task.

For the measurement of the body fat various skin-fold callipers have been devised like the Harpender and the Lange Calipers. These are relatively inexpensive. The procedure is painless if done correctly and can yield a good estimate of percentage body fat. This technique has a limitation that if performed by untrained people the skin folds may not be obtained easily and accurately.

The measurement of skin-fold thickness can be carried out at triceps, sub-scapular, biceps and super iliac.

1. *Triceps:* This is done at a point equidistant from tip of acromion and the olecranon.
2. *Sub-scapular:* Just below the tip of the inferior angle of scapula.
3. *Bicep:* At the mid point of the muscle with the arm hanging vertically.
4. *Super iliac:* Over the iliac crest in the mid axillary line.

In case of difficulties to measure the skin-fold thickness at four sites the most appropriate site for measurement could be the single measurement over triceps. The measurement of triceps should be less than 85 to 90 percentile for the age.

5. Ponderal Index

It is the ratio of height to the cube root of weight. It is denoted by PI.

$PI = ht\ (inches) / \sqrt[3]{wt(lbs)}$, A PI <13, indicates obesity.

6. Broca's Index

This is the method for quick measurement of ideal body weight for an average individual. This index indicates higher ideal body weight than those indicated by other standard tables.

$$\boxed{Ht\ (cm) - 100 = ideal\ wt\ (kg)}$$

7. Corpulence Index

This refers to the ratio of weight of the person to the desired weight of the person. The ratio exceeding greater than 1.2 is indicative of obesity.

8. Lean Body Mass

To calculate the lean body mass, measurement of the percentage of body water is required. It is estimated by using titrated water or antipyrine.

% body fat = 100 − [% body water / 0.732]

The average water content of LBM is 73.2 per cent.

Dilution Method: Water soluble compound is injected into the blood stream and the extent to which the compound is diluted can give an appropriate amount of lean tissue in the body.

Since potassium is by and large found in the lean tissues of the body, measurement of naturally occurring isotope of potassium can be done to determine the amount of lean tissue in the body.

Tanita BIA

Tanita has developed a simplified version of BIA that uses leg-to-leg bioimpedance analysis. In this system, two footpad electrode (pressure contact) are incorporated to the platform of precision electronic scale. The person's measurements are taken while in a standing position with the electrodes in contact with the bare feet. The body fat monitor or analyser automatically measures weight followed by impedance. A computer software (microprocessor) imbedded in the product uses the measured impedance, the subject's gender, height fitness level and in some cases age and the weight to determine body fat percentage based on the *equation.*

Total Body Electrical Conductivity (TOBEC)

This method is based on the principle that lean tissues are better conductivity of electricity than fat. Here the person is made to lie in a cylinder that generates a very low electromagnetic field. The strength of the field depends on the electrolytes found in a person's body water. In 10 seconds TOBEC makes 10 conductivity readings that estimate lean body mass. Although very accurate, its use is limited due to high cost of the equipment.

9. Body Density Measurement

It can be assessed by underwater weighing and the proportion of adipose tissue can also be measured.

Underwater weighing is a standard method for estimating the body fat. It is usually considered for verifying the results of measuring body fat by other methods. The subject is first weighed on dry land; next he or she is submerged in water and exhales completely; then his or her weight is measured. The less the person weighs under water compared to the weight on dry land, the higher the percentage of body fat.

Accurate value of percentage body fat can be calculated using appropriate formulas. This method has a limitation as it is expensive and cannot be used for people who do not swim or who are disabled.

The density of normal weight subjects is known to be 1.0629 g/ml at 37°C and the density of obese tissue is 0.947 g/ml at 37°C.

Bioelectrical Impedance Analysis (BIA)

Since fat is a poor conductor of electricity, and water and muscles are good conductors, body fat content can be estimated by determining how quickly electrical current passes from the ankle to the wrist.

The equipment used to measure bioelectrical impedance analysis is portable, and the test is easy to perform and is painless. This method gives fairly accurate results for average individuals. It should be conducted in individuals with an empty bladder, those who had been fasting overnight and in those who have performed strenuous exercise. The limitation is that the equipment is expensive. Variations in the hydration status of individuals may affect electrical conductivity and may give inaccurate results.

Magnetic Resonance Imaging (MRI)

MRI and CT or CAT scans provide similar results. Using this technology, a person's body fat and muscle mass can be photographed when exposed to a magnetic field (or, in the case of CAT scans, to radiation). Based on the volume of fat and muscle observed, total fat and muscle content can be determined. These methods give a precise estimation of fat and muscle mass. It is expensive and mostly used for research purposes.

10. Saggital Diameter

Sjostrom and colleagues have developed this measurement to estimate abdominal and visceral fat. This is obtained by making the individual lie flat on the plain surface. A bubble gauge is then placed on top of the flat surface which can then be aligned with a vertical measurement of the distance between the abdomen and the surface on which the subject is lying.

Estimating the Energy Requirements

This is basically a three step process:
1. Determining the energy needed for RMR of the body;
2. Physical activity;
3. Thermic effect of food.

Resting Metabolic Rate Based on Body Weight

Body weight	(kg)	40	50	57	64	70	77	84	91	100
	(lb)	88	110	125	140	155	170	185	200	220
					Kcalories per 24 hours					
Male Age (yr)										
10-18		1351	1526	1648	1771	1876	1998	2121	2243	2401
18-30		1291	1444	1551	1658	1750	1857	1964	2071	2209
30-60		1343	1459	1540	1621	1691	1772	1853	1935	2039
> 60		1027	1162	1256	1351	1423	1526	1621	1716	1837
Female Age (yr)										
10-18		1234	1356	1441	1527	1600	1685	1771	1856	1966
18-30		1084	1231	1334	1437	1525	1628	1731	1833	1966
30-60		1177	1264	1325	1386	1438	1499	1560	1621	1699
> 60		1016	1121	1195	1268	1331	1404	1478	1552	1646

The body derives energy from foods for muscular activity, growth, tissue repair and maintenance. Energy is also required to chemically process nutrients and to maintain body temperature. These needs for energy are categorised into three categories:

(a) Basal metabolism;

(b) Physical activity;

(c) Dietary thermogenesis.

Basal Metabolism

Activities that the body performs while at rest, work, or play make up the maximum of calories needed by the body and that usually ranges from 60 to 80 percent. These activities sustain basal metabolism that normally comprise of processes such as breathing, the beating of the heart, the maintenance of body temperature, growth, and the transport of nutrients to, and waste products out of cells. The basal metabolic processes use up the energy and does not require any special effort on our part. They are continuous activities that the body must perform to maintain life. The energy needed to carry out basal metabolic functions is evaluated when the body is in a state of complete physical and emotional rest.

The calories needed for basal metabolism based on sex and weight can be estimated as below. Other factors, particular.y physical activity level, muscle mass, height and genetic traits, also affect how efficiently the body uses calories for basal metabolism.

For men: Multiply body weight in kg by 24.2
For women: Multiply body weight in kg by 22

Thus a man who weighs 77 kg needs approximately 77 × 24.2, or 1863 calories per day for basal metabolic processes. A 61 kg woman needs 61 × 22 or 1342 calories.

The energy required for BMR is estimated in the above manner is an approximation and may be 10 to 20% lower or higher than the true number of calories.

Physical Activity

The energy required for physical activity normally depends on how active a person is. It usually accounts for the second highest amount of energy we use up.

The energy cost of supporting a sedentary lifestyle (see table below) is about 30% of the number of calories needed for basal metabolism. Moderately active person requires approximately 50% and a very active individual requires approximately 75% of the calories needed for basal metabolism. A moderately active person requiring 1800 calories a day for basal metabolism, for example, would require about 900 calories (1800 X 0.50) for physical activity.

Table: Energy Cost in Terms of % of Basal Metabolism for Individuals with Varying Physical Activity

Activity Level	% of BM Calories
Inactive: Sitting most of the day, less than two hours of moving about slowly or standing.	30%
Average: Sitting most of the day, walking or standing two to four hours, but no strenuous activity.	50%
Active: Physically active four or more hours each day; little sitting or standing, some physically strenuous activities.	75%

Dietary Thermogenesis

A portion of the body's energy expenditure is used for a variety of physical and metabolic processes such as digesting foods, absorbing and utilising nutrients, and transporting nutrients into cells. Some of the energy involved in such activities is liberated in the form of heat. These processes are referred to as the energy cost of dietary thermogenesis. Calories spent for dietary thermogenesis are predicted as 10% of the sum of basal metabolic and physical activity calories.

E.g. A person's basal metabolic need is 1800 calories and 900 calories are required for usual activity: 1800 calories + 900 calories = 2700 calories. Calories expended for dietary thermogenesis would be approximately 10% of 2700 calories or 270 calories.

Therefore summing up the calories required per day would be 1800 + 900 + 270, or 2970. Although the caloric level calculated will not be exactly right, it should provide a good estimate of the total caloric need.

Energy expenditure can also be determined by multiplying the RMR with the factor that is derived from various activity level.

Since the RMR of individuals differs with age, sex and body weight the RMR of individuals can be calculated using the following table:

Adopted from: National Research Council, RDA, Wed Washington DC, National Academy of Services, 1989.

Factors for estimating energy requirements for various activities in relation to RMR.

Level of Activity	Activity Factor/ Unit Time of Activity
Resting (Sleeping, reclining)	BMR × 1.0
Very light (Seated, standing activities, painting, driving, laboratory work, typing, sewing, ironing, cooking, playing cards, playing musical instruments)	BMR × 1.5
Light (Walking on a level surface (2.5-3 miles/hour), garage work, carpentry, house cleaning, golf)	BMR × 2.5
Moderate (Walking 3.5-4 miles/hour, weeding, carrying load, cycling, skipping, tennis and dancing)	BMR × 5.0
Heavy (Walking with load uphill, tree felling, heavy manual digging, basketball, climbing, football)	BMR × 7

Calculating the energy expenditure for a college going student (female) of age 21 years weighing 64 kg.

According to the table:
1. The RMR of this girl is 1437 kcal / 24 hours = 60 kcal per hour.
2. The energy required for different activities calculated using the RMR factor is:
   (a) Rest   8 hours × 60 × 1   = 480
   (b) Very light activity   11 hours × 60 × 1.5 = 990
   (c) Light activity   3 hours × 60 × 2.5 = 450

Energy requirement for thermic effect of food is about 10% of daily energy intake.

$$= 1928 + 10\% \text{ thermic effect} = 2113$$

Thus the estimated total energy expenditure for the girl
$$= RMR + activity + TEF$$

Recent Advances

Body fat content can also be assessed by ultrasound, magnetic resonance spectroscopy, neuron activation analysis, and dual energy X-ray absorptiometer (DXA). These methods are highly technical and expensive, however, and are used infrequently because of their cost or lack of availability.

5
Complications of Obesity

Obesity invites various complications which are life threatening. Some of these are listed below:

1. Heart disease and strokes
2. Diabetes mellitus
3. Hypertension
4. Hypercholestrolemia
5. Gall bladder disease (Cholelithiasis)
6. Dyslipidemia
7. Certain types of cancers
8. Sleep apnea and other respiratory problems
9. Osteoarthritis
10. Emotional disturbances and social stigmatisation
11. Reduced fertility and pregnancy complications
12. Restricted mobility
13. Mechanical disability
14. Gallstones
15. Fatty liver
16. Skin disorders
17. Other comorbidities

1. Heart Disease and Stroke

The risk of cardiovascular disease increases significantly when the BMI exceeds 25.0 kg per m² and most dramatically as the BMI level surpass 30 kg per m². Longitudinal studies suggests that obesity is an important independent risk factor for CHD (Coronary Heart Disease) related morbidity and mortality. The Framingham Heart Study ranked body weight as the third most important predictor of CHD in males after age and dyslipidemia. The Asian Indians have the highest rates of CHD of any ethnic group studies, despite the fact that nearly half of these populations are life long vegetarians. This can also be attributed to high triglyceride, low HDL, hyperinsulinaemia and abdominal obesity.

Severe obesity can lead to an abnormal lipid profile including high circulating levels of LDL cholesterol and low levels of HDL cholesterol which may culminate into artherosclerosis. Build up of the fatty streaks in the arteries along with platelets deposition can give rise to clots in the blood vessels that may block the blood flow in the brain resulting into a stroke.

2. Diabetes Mellitus

Insulin maintains the level of blood sugar (glucose). When there is too much fat in the body the body becomes resistant to insulin and this results in high blood sugar levels. Obesity is an important risk factor for diabetes mellitus. The prevalence of overweight and obesity in the diabetic adults in USA was found to be 67% and 46% respectively. A study carried out in Iran, showed that out of 85 patients with type 2 diabetes mellitus 46% were found to be overweight and obese indicating a strong association of obesity with diabetes mellitus.

3. Hypertension

Like all other tissues, the fatty tissue requires oxygen and blood nutrients for survival. In obesity, there is more of fatty tissue and hence there will be increase in the amount of blood circulating through the body, which results in greater pressure on the walls of the arteries resulting in high blood pressure. Overweight and obese men and women are known to have a higher degree of hypertension when compared to their normal counterparts. The NIDDK Weight-Control Information Network has reported that in USA 41.9% obese men and 37.8% obese women suffered from moderate degree of hypertension when compared to 14.4% men and 15.2% women having normal weights.

4. Hypercholestrolemia

Obesity is known to cause high blood cholesterol in both men and women. A study reported by NIDDK Weight-Control Information Network revealed that in USA 22% obese men and 27% obese women suffered from high blood cholesterol when compared to 13% men and 13.4% women having normal weight. A great number of overweight women (30.5%) in USA suffer from high blood cholesterol.

5. Gall Bladder Disease (Cholelithiasis)

There is an increase in the amount of the cholesterol synthesised by the body each day by about 20 mg for each kilogram of adipose tissue. An increase of 10 kg in adipose tissue mass results in increased production and excretion of cholesterol to a level, which is equivalent to the value of cholesterol present in one egg. Hence with advancement in age and severity of obesity, there is an increased risk of gall bladder disease due to a rise in the excretion of biliary cholesterol. In the Nurses Health Study, there was a gradual increase in the incidence rate of cholelithiasis with increase in BMI to a level of 30 kg/m² and a very steep increase when the BMI was higher than 30 kg/m².

6. Dyslipidemia

Obese people in general tend to have an elevation of fasting plasma total cholesterol, triglyceride and a reduction in plasma high density lipoprotein cholesterol (HDL-C). Plasma LDL-C are slightly elevated or normal in obese persons but the number of small densed atherogenic LDL particles is usually increased particularly in patients with insulin-resistant syndrome associated with abdominal obesity.

Very Low Density Lipoprotein

Central obesity and hyperinsulinemia accompanying insulin resistance are known to produce excess of VLDL in liver which is triglyceride rich. Enhanced lipolytic activity of visceral adipocyte may cause an increased free fatty acid flux to the liver and stimulate VLDL secretion. In addition the lipoprotein lipase levels are decreased resulting in slower clearance of VLDL and a reduced production of HDL particles. This alteration in VLDL metabolism can lead to production of smaller denser LDL particles.

High Total Cholesterol

According to NHANES III the relationship of high total cholesterol has shown that at each BMI level the prevalence of high blood cholesterol is greater in women than in men. Total cholesterol are known to be higher in persons with predominant abdominal obesity.

High Triglyceride

A significant association of triglyceride levels with BMI has been reported in both cross-sectional as well as longitudinal studies for both sexes and in all age groups.

Low High Density Lipoprotein Cholesterol (HDL)
Cross-sectional studies have reported that HDL cholesterol is lower in men and women with higher BMI. Longitudinal studies found that the changes in BMI are associated with changes in HDL cholesterol. A BMI change of 1 unit is associated with HDL cholesterol change of 1.1 mg/dL for young adults and an HDL cholesterol change of 0.69 mg/dL for young adult women.

7. Certain Types of Cancers
Being overweight can result into various types of cancers like the incidence of endometrial and postmenopausal breast cancers in women, prostate cancer in men, colon cancer and gall bladder cancer. The risk of endometrial cancer increases upto 20 fold in most obese women and in an American Cancer Society Prospective study a four fold increase in mortality was reported in women with BMI > 35, whereas men with BMI >31 have a 20 to 30 percent increase in prostrate cancer related mortality. Men and women with BMI>35 have increased mortality from colon cancers. A recent study found that people whose BMI was 40 or more had death rates from cancer that were 52 percent higher for men and 62 percent higher for women than rates for normal weight men and women. Overweight and obesity could account for 14 percent of cancer deaths among men and 20 percent among women in the US. In both men and women, higher BMI is associated with higher death rates from cancers of the esophagus, colon and rectum, liver, gall bladder, pancreas, and kidney. The same trend applies to cancers of the stomach and prostate in men and cancers of the breast, uterus, cervix, and ovaries in women. Almost half of postmenopausal women diagnosed with breast cancer have a BMI $\geq$ 29.19. In postmenopausal women with BMI>35, the mortality ratio due to breast cancer has been reported as 1.53. In one study (the Nurses' Health Study),

women gaining more than 20 pounds from age 18 to midlife doubled their risk of breast cancer, compared to women whose weight remained stable.

8. Sleep Apnea and Other Respiratory Problems

As people gain weight many complain that they feel tired all the time and have problems obtaining a restful sleep. Problems with sleep may be indicative of a severe condition called Pickwickian Syndrome, or sleep apnea. This occurs because of more fat in the neck region and narrow airways which cause the upper airway to become blocked during sleep.

For people with this problem, it becomes progressively more difficult to breathe (especially at night) as their weight increases. These people typically snore severely and have episodes of apnea, sometimes upto one minute at a time.

During these non-breathing periods, heart rhythms may become very irregular, which can lead to a fatal heart attack. Frequently, people with sleep apnea transiently awaken when they resume breathing. This may occur dozens of times per night, causing the afflicted individual to feel tired the next day. Sometimes these individuals will fall asleep while sitting in meetings or driving. Sleep apnea is a very serious complication of obesity and requires professional medical attention. The best method of treatment is losing weight, however, other measures are available to improve the breathing process and help prevent the heart irregularities that frequently complicate this condition.

People with lesser degrees of obesity may also have problems in sleeping. Sleep disturbances are also associated with anxiety and depression. Depression is not just feeling blue for a day, but is the result of actual chemical changes that take place in the brain, causing profound episodes of sadness, crying and loss of energy. Depression is a medical condition that requires medical treatment. There are effective non-addicting medications available if depression is complicating obesity.

9. Osteoarthritis

Excess weight in the body gives more stress on the joints, particularly the hips, knees and lower back. It causes more wear and tear of the joints. Such disorders increase the pressure on the joints. This results in wearing away of cartilages protecting the joints resulting in osteoarthritis. Adipose tissue also produces substances i.e. cytokines which destroy normal cartilages of joints. Some obese children are also known to develop orthopedic problems such as slipped capital femoral epiphysis, tibial torsion and bowed legs and symptoms of weight stress in the joints of the lower extremities (Sriram, 2001). A study of twins found that with every kg increase in body weight was associated with increased risk of radiographic features of osteoarthritis at the knee and at Carpometacarpal joint.

In contrast to weight gain weight loss is also associated with decreased risk of osteoarthritis. In a study of 800 women a decrease in BMI of 2 kg / m^2 or more in the preceding 10 years decreased the odds for developing osteoarthritis by over 50%.

10. Emotional Disturbances and Social Stigmatisation

Obese people are often teased and ostracised. They frequently find themselves isolated socially from their peers. Such people also experience discrimination in college admissions, job markets and in matrimonial success. It becomes a challenge for them to dress up for social gatherings as they find difficult to wear the clothes that are in vogue and appeal to the general mass.

11. Reduced Fertility and Pregnancy Complications

Obesity during pregnancy increases the risk of death both in baby and the mother. There is also a risk of getting high blood pressure and gestational diabetes. Moreover obese women during pregnancy may have complications of labour and delivery.

Infants born to obese women are likely to be overweight and may have to undergo Ceasarean delivery that can be a risk to a brain damage.

12. Restricted Mobility

Obesity leads to physical impairments which include difficulty in climbing stairs, walking in a crowded area, or sitting on vehicles etc. which results into restricted mobility.

Severe obesity reduces mobility and freedom of movement making people more accident-prone. Excess weight hampers the most basic tasks that the body needs to perform such as walking and breathing.

13. Mechanical Disability

In obese people there is extra load on the skeleton. Since the bones have to bear excess weight such people usually experience complications like flat foot, osteoarthritis. The mechanical action of the muscle is impaired as they get infilterated with fat.

14. Gallstones

Gallstones are formed from excessive precipitation of cholesterol and when they grow in size and number they may disrupt the flow of bile from gall bladder into the duct. Obesity is a strong risk factor for gallstones because researchers have reported that obese people produce high amounts of cholesterol than the normal and this leads to the production of bile containing more cholesterol than it can dissolve. People who are obese have large gall bladders that do not empty normally or completely

Rapid weight reduction increases the risk of developing gallstones. Moreover the persons undergoing very low calorie diet increases the risk of developing gallstones. This is because dieting may cause a shift in the balance of bile salts and cholesterol and increase the levels of cholesterol and decrease the levels of bile salts. Continuing with such diet for a long time decreases the gall bladder contractions. If gall bladder does not contract often to empty the bile gallstones can form.

15. Fatty Liver

This condition, which was known to occur in older people who had a long history of alcohol consumption, is now making its appearance in obese children with syndrome X. Such children are known to consume large quantities of very high fat and carbohydrate diet consisting mainly of bread, butter, chips, ice creams, burgers, cheese, etc.

16. Skin Disorders

Obese people are more prone to skin disorders than the non- obese especially if deep skin folds are present. These include heat rash, intertrigo, monilial dermatitis and acanthosis nigricans (a condition that may be a marker for type 2 diabetes.)

Hirsutism in women may result from increased production of testosterone which is often associated with visceral obesity. Stretch marks are common and reflect the tension on the skin from the expanding deposits of subcutaneous fat. Venous statis is also increased in obese people.

17. Other Co-morbidities

Obese patients may also have edema, gastro esophageal reflux, urinary stress incontinence, idiopathic intracranial hypertension. They may also suffer from diseases of lower extremities, impaired cell mediated immunity, obstetric complications including toxemia, hypertension. They are also prone to longer labour, increased liability to accidents and increased morbidity in acute pancreatitis.

Mortality

Most studies show an increase in mortality rate associated with obesity (BMI ≥ 30). Obese individuals have a 50 to 100 percent increased risk of death from all causes, compared with normal-weight individuals (BMI 20–25). Most of the increased risk is due to cardiovascular causes. Life expectancy of a moderately obese person could be shortened by 2 to 5 years. White men between 20 and 30 years old with a BMI ≥ 45 could shorten their life expectancy by 13 years; white women in the same category could lose up to 8 years of life. Young African American men with a BMI ≥ 45 could lose up to 20 years of life; African American women, up to 5.

The Nurses Health Study has reported that the risk of death rose progressively in women with BMI above 29 kg/m². Aerobics Center Longitudinal Study which had 25,714 men as subjects and was followed from 1-10 years revealed that the all cause mortality and cardiovascular mortality was higher in men with the BMI > 30 kg/m² and lowest in those with BMI between 18.5 and 24.9 kg/m² with men having a BMI of 25 to 29.9 kg/m² falling in between.

6
Management of Obesity

The method of dealing with obesity depends on the BMI, the overall health conditions and the individual's motivation to lose weight. Even a reduction of 5 kg of weight can reduce the chances of a person developing several complications of obesity.

It is an ideal situation for an obese individual to achieve a normal BMI (18.5-25) but difficult to achieve. However attempts should be made to reach it as near as possible.

Its treatment includes a combination of diet, exercise, behaviour and motivation and sometimes using the weight loss drugs. In extreme conditions surgery is considered to be a mode of treatment. But in the majority of cases, a blend of diet and exercise is an ideal combination and more effective.

The treatment for obesity is challenging and a complicated issue. What works for one person may not be effective for another. Professional counselling by an experienced well-qualified dietician can help you achieve weight loss more successfully.

Strategies for Management of Obesity

1. Assessment of excess weight
2. Willingness and commitment by the subject to reduce weight
3. Estimation of energy requirement

4. Setting realistic goals for weight loss
5. Behaviour and motivation therapy
6. Dietary modifications
7. Careful exercise plan
8. Compliance on the part of subject
9. Record the progress
10. Deviation analysis in case of weight loss failure and counselling for the deviations

The other methods less commonly employed for treating obesity are;
1. Psycho therapy
2. Drug therapy
3. Surgery
4. Gastric balloons and jaw wiring

1. Assessment of Excess Weight

It can be calculated by various methods explained in chapter 4.

However, the most accepted and practical method is calculating the Body Mass Index followed by determination of excess body weight after comparing with the standard body weight for the said age and height or referring to the nomogram for BMI.

2. Willingness and Commitment by the Subject to Reduce Weight

Having a committed attitude on the part of the subject is the critical first step towards successful weight loss plan. The subject should not take advantage of the interest he/she has in losing weight temporarily. They should also not jump into a weight loss programme when there is a mood swing. Such an approach will lead to disappointment for there is no magic cure for treating obesity. It is a long term process and success will come your way only through a strong determination to lose weight and following the diet and exercise plan strictly.

3. **Estimation of Energy Requirement**

   As per chapter 4

4. **Setting Realistic Goals for Weight Loss**

The World Health Organisation (WHO) has recommended a safe upper limit of 1.0 kg weight loss per week for overweight but otherwise normal individuals. However, losing 2.0 to 3.0 kg a month is attainable through careful eating and exercise programme and can be considered as the most sensible goal. One way to keep a check on calorie consumption is to maintain a diet diary for a week and to determine the weight loss attained. A diet plan can then be made which provides about 500 calories less per day than presently being consumed. As long as the individual is exercising, one can lose around 0.5 to 1.0 kg of weight per week. Fast weight-loss programmes actually make it more difficult to lose weight because they slow your metabolism. As a result you regain the lost weight.

Most people trying to lose weight focus on just that one goal: weight loss. However, it is important to look at the process of weight loss wherein one needs to also focus on the dietary and exercise changes that will lead to that long-term weight change. Successful weight managers are those who select two or three goals at a time that the subjects are willing to take on, and those that meet the following criteria of useful goals:

Effective goals are (1) specific; (2) attainable; and (3) forgiving (less than perfect). "Exercise more" is a commendable ideal, but it is not specific. "Walk five kilometers everyday" is specific and measurable, but is it attainable if you 'are just starting out?" "Walk 30 minutes every day" is more attainable, but what happens if you are held up at work one day and there is a thunderstorm during your walking time another day? "Walk 30 minutes, five days each week" is specific, attainable, and forgiving. In short, a great goal!

5. Behaviour and Motivation Therapy

The degree to which a person is motivated and is ready to implement the weight management plan is an important factor in weight loss programme. Changing overall lifestyle and adopting a positive lifestyle, valuing self-motivation and setting goals is an essential component of long term weight loss. Support in terms of family, friends and the physician is important which helps the person to reduce weight.

Behaviour modification for beginners and maintaining an exercise programme.

1. Start slowly – Instead of planning to run three miles a day five times a week, plan to start with a 20 minutes walk three days per week.
2. Make it fun – Choose activities you enjoy and find a partner with whom to exercise.
3. Set specific attainable goals – ' I will walk for 20 minutes on Mondays, Wednesday and Fridays.
4. Make it convenient – Plan to walk early in the morning, during your lunch hour at work or after dinner.
5. Record your programme – Keep a record of your activity so that you can check your programme and keep yourself motivated.
6. Reward yourself – Plan to reward yourself when you succeed at your goal. (a new book or a movie)

An essential component for long term weight loss is changing the overall lifestyle. It means changing how a person thinks, acts and feels, changing the way a person views food and exercises, valuing self-motivation, setting goals and other positive lifestyle enhancements.

Behaviour therapy constitutes those strategies, based on learning principles such as reinforcement that provides tools for overcoming barriers to compliance with dietary therapy or increased physical activity. E.g. **behaviour modification technique** includes self-monitoring, stimulus control, cognitive restructuring, stress management and social support.

Self-monitoring

It refers to observing and recording some aspect of your behaviour, such as calorie intake, servings of fruits and vegetables, exercise sessions, medication usage, etc., or an outcome of these behaviours, such as weight. Self-monitoring of a behaviour can be used at times when you are not sure how you are doing, and at times when you want the behaviour to improve. Self-monitoring of a behaviour usually changes the behaviour in the desired direction and can produce " real-time" records for review by you and your health care provider. For example, keeping a record of your exercise can let you and your provider know quickly how you are doing, and when the record shows that your exercise is increasing, you will be encouraged to keep it up. Some patients find that specific self-monitoring forms make it easier, while others prefer to use their own recording system.

While you may or may not wish to weigh yourself frequently while losing weight, regular monitoring of your weight will be essential to help you maintain your lower weight. When keeping a record of your weight, a graph may be more informative than a list of your weights. When weighing yourself and keeping a weight graph or table, however, remember that one day's diet and exercise patterns will not have a measurable effect on your fat weight the next day. Today's weight is not a true measure of how well you followed your programme yesterday, because your body's water weight will change much more from day-to-day than will your fat weight, and water changes are often the result of things that have nothing to do with your weight-management efforts.

Stimulus (cue) Control
It involves learning what social or environmental cues seem to encourage undesired eating, and then changing those cues. For example, you may learn from reflection or from self-monitoring records that you are more likely to overeat while watching television, or whenever treats are on display by the office coffee pot, or when around a certain friend. You might then try to associate eating with the cue (do not eat while watching television), avoid or eliminate the cue (leave coffee room immediately after pouring coffee), or change the circumstances surrounding the cue (plan to meet with a friend in non-food settings). In general, visible and accessible food items are often cues for unplanned eating.

Cognitive Restructuring
Changing the way you go about eating can make it easier to eat less without feeling deprived. It takes 15 or more minutes for your brain to get the message you have been fed. Slowing the rate of eating can allow satiety (fullness) signals to begin to develop by the end of the meal. Eating lots of vegetables can also make you feel fuller. Another trick is to use smaller plates so that moderate portions do not appear meager. Changing your eating schedule, or setting one, can be helpful, especially if you tend to skip, or delay, meals and overeat later.

How Avoidable Calories in the Meals Can Increase Unknowingly:

1. While making tea: Make a habit of measuring sugar and milk before adding. Standardise your cup of tea with low sugar/ sugar free and skimmed milk.

2. Do not add shortening to a dough for chappati/*bhakhri* and serve them hot. Tasty parathas can be made with just one teaspoon of fat instead of two tablespoons normally used.
3. Always measure oil while seasoning the vegetables/dals. For a family of four approximate two teaspoons of oil should be sufficient to make a palatable dish.
4. Do not add fat (pure ghee) into rice/*khichdi*.
5. Certain foods like *dhokla, idada, handwa, dhebhra, patra*, etc., can taste good without added oil when taken hot.
6. Dosas made in non-stick pan require fat as low as 2 grams per piece.
7. Boiled potatoes are healthier than shallow fried/deep fried.
8. Enjoy cooking your meals yourself rather than buying ready to eat high calorie foods. It helps you to consume a meal which is balanced in quantity and quality.

6. Dietary Modifications

It is a common mode of treatment for all obese individuals. The obese should be educated regarding his/her nutritional adequacy, meal size, frequency and timings. The treatment should consist of reducing the weight by burning excess fat of the body. In order to get quick results many people follow crash dieting. This is not an appropriate method and should be considered as advocated by fools. A systematic approach of obesity management leads to slow but steady reduction in fat, which is usually recommended by dieticians.

Principle

Low calorie, low fat, adequate proteins, vitamins and minerals, liberal amount of fluid and good fibre diet is recommended.

To give a correct dietary treatment the dietician should find out the extra weight of the person. Depending on the height and age the ideal weight of the person can be calculated by using the height-weight table (Appendix No 1a). The excess weight is now calculated by subtracting the ideal weight from the present weight. Considering the excess fat the dietician would decide the rate of burning the fat by prescribing an appropriate diet and exercise plan.

Energy

In an obese person, the main target is to reduce the energy-dense foods. The desirable calorie intake for the person undergoing a weight loss regimen is given in 20 kcal/kg of ideal body weight. For e.g. if the ideal body weight is 50 kg then an individual needs to take 1000 calorie diet (50 × 20) per day. A sample diet providing 1000 calories is given in the table.

Research all over the world has shown that obese subjects consume significantly more total calories than the non-obese subjects (14, 39). The desirable calorie intake for the person undergoing a weight loss regimen is already explained above.

A Calorie is a Calorie Whether it Comes from Fat or Fruit

Some misconceptions need to be clarified with regards to popular beliefs amongst individual undergoing weight loss programme with inadequate knowledge about the calorie content of foods. For e.g. rice has more calories than wheat. In fact 100g of rice (3 cups cooked) and 100g of wheat flour (5 medium-size chappaties i.e. 20g per chappati) have similar calorie content. Similarly there is a belief that ghee has more calories than oil. The fact is that 100g of ghee or oil contains similar amount of calories (900 calories).

Also, potatoes are rich source of nutrients specially the vitamins and need not be totally avoided from meals of individual undergoing weight loss. They are best eaten when boiled and fried in small quantities.

Protein
Proteins are essential for tissue repair and specific dynamic action. About 1 gram protein per kg of ideal body weight is recommended.

Fat
Fats are considered as concentrated source of energy and hence should be taken in limited amount. The amount of fat taken should be such that it provides only taste and satiety to the diet. No more than 20 grams of fat per day is necessary for fulfilling the requirements of essential fatty acids and for the absorption of fat soluble vitamins. Ideally 15 to 20% calories should come from fat. Since 1 g of fat gives 9 kcal, 15-20% calories would mean on a 1000 kcal diet 16-22 grams of fat per day can be taken.

Carbohydrates
Simple carbohydrates like those present in jams, syrups and fruit juices contains high amount of carbohydrates and also do not give bulk to the diet. Such food items should generally be avoided. To produce satiety and to have regular bowel movements carbohydrates like those present in green leafy vegetables, fruits etc., should be prescribed.

Carbohydrates should contribute 60 to 70 per cent of total calorie mainly in the form of complex carbohydrates consisting of high amounts of soluble fibre that can come from whole grain cereals, pulses, fruits that are not skinned and salad vegetables, other vegetables etc.

Vitamins and Minerals
A balanced diet consisting of foods from all the food groups generally can provide all the necessary vitamins and minerals

that are required by the body even on a low calorie (1000 kcal) diet. If correct diet is followed then one does not need to take vitamin supplements on a weight-reducing diet.

Fluids

Fluids can be taken liberally. A glass of water before meal helps to cut down the food intake. It gives the feeling of fullness. Minimum of 6-8 glasses of water per day can prevent a person from eating large quantities of food.

Fiber

The diet should contain good amount of fiber-rich foods like green leafy vegetables, fruits, vegetable salads, pulses, whole grains, cereals, legumes etc. Fiber gives satiety and helps in regulating the bowel movements. Fibers promotes chewing which decreases the rate of ingestion. It also reduces the blood cholesterol. Fiber limits energy intake by lowering a food's density and allowing time for appetite control signals to occur before large amounts of energy have been consumed.

In order to incorporate variety in the diet one can choose low calorie food items from the low calorie/low fat recipes described in Chapter 9.

7. Careful Exercise Plan

Exercise along with the dietary management is an ideal combination and should be an integral part in the weight management programme. It decreases the abdominal fat and increases the cardiorespiratory fitness.

Exercise helps in the following ways:
1. In reducing weight
2. In increasing strength
3. In increasing endurance

Exercising not only burns calories and compensates for the slower metabolism that comes with eating less but it also makes you healthier. A daily walk is a great first step. Then, try swimming, dancing, jogging, or anything that gets you going. Or just make small changes in your daily routine, like taking the stairs when you can instead of the lift. The following table shows how one should carry out different exercises so as to burn 100 calories with respect to various activities.

Energy expenditure
How to burn 100 calories?

Activity	Time
Dusting	40 mins
Cleaning car	23 mins
Mopping floor	23 mins
Ironing clothes	43 mins
Tidying your room	43 mins
Gardening	1 hour and 7 mins
Dancing	23 mins
Trekking	17 mins
Brisk walking	25 mins
Cycling	25 mins
Pull ups, push ups and sit ups	12.5 mins
Weight lifting	34 mins
Yoga and stretching	25 mins
Aerobics	17 mins
Climbing stairs	20 mins
Jogging	14 mins
Badminton	23 mins
Cricket	20 mins
Golf	23 mins
Table tennis	25 mins
Lawn tennis	14 mins
Swimming	17 mins

The regularity in the physical exercises is of utmost importance in successful weight reduction programme.

Some more ways of reducing weight include intercourse, yoga (*Paschimottasan, Bhujangasan, Chakrasan, Dhanurasan, Nari Shodh Pranayam.*)

> It is also a good idea to build strength training into your workouts. The less muscle you have, the harder it is to lose weight and keep it off. Here is why: muscle is metabolically active; it takes energy, in the form of calories, to sustain it. Fat is not, and it does not. So the more muscle you have, the more calories you burn, even at rest. Two or three 30-minute weight-lifting sessions each week will make a big difference in your body composition and, therefore, in the number of calories you burn each day.

One should generally undertake the exercise that does not increase one's heart rate beyond 90% but >60% of the maximum heart rate of that individual.

Maximum heart rate = 220 − age

If the age of the individual is 45 years

The maximum heart rate = 220 − 45 = 175 beats

Now 60% of maximum 175 × 0.6 = 105 beat/min

90% of maximum 175 × 0.9 = 158 beats/min

Thus, one should exercise at a heart rate of at least 105 beats/minute and not more than 158 beats/minute.

Precautions for Safe Exercising

1. Before beginning any exercise programme one must check with their physicians to make sure that they are fit enough to take the exercise plan.
2. A safe well-lit location must be sought for instead of late evenings or early mornings.
3. One must always begin the exercise with "warm-up" to increase the blood flow to muscles. This includes stretching and some easy walking or jogging.
4. Avoid exercising in extreme environmental conditions. During exercising heat is produced by the body, which is removed through sweat. But in extremely hot and humid environments the sweat does evaporate fast and cools the body rather slowly whereas in the cold weather

due to heavy clothing the evaporation of sweat becomes difficult. Therefore it is advisable to wear light-coloured cotton clothes that supports sweat absorption or evaporation so that the body temperature can rapidly turn to normal.

8. Compliance on the Part of the Subject

The compliance with the non-surgical treatment of obesity varies widely. In a study conducted in a weight-reducing clinic, successful targeted weight loss could be achieved in the range of 75 to 100 % in male and female subjects. Some of the reasons attributed for not achieving 100% success were low motivation on part of the subjects, strong resistance to dietary change, expectations of some subjects for a dramatic weight reduction and some were hard pressed for time and were satisfied with the weight loss that was achieved. In this health clinic the drop out rate was 10.8% and was found to be more in females than in males. Maximum drop out rate was seen in females in the age group of 42-49 years. In case of men the reasons given for not complying with the weight loss programme was their inability to keep to their appointments. Other reasons for poor compliance were business dinners, eating away from home, acidity and mental hunger. The subjects who complied maximum with the weight loss programme developed a positive self-image.

9. Record the Progress

It is important to record the progress of weight loss by maintaining a diet diary. Weight should be taken fortnightly and recorded in the diary. Along with this the special efforts made to avoid high calorie foods should also be recorded. Conditions that trigger overeating should be noted and care should be taken to avoid them.

10. Deviation Analysis in Case of Weight Loss Failure and Counselling for the Deviations

Any deviations in the prescribed diet should be brought to the notice of the counsellor and should be worked upon in order to achieve the targeted weight loss. In a study on 270 clients with 173 females and 67 males enrolled at weight-reducing clinic reported a strong resistance in their attitudes towards a prescribed diet which reflected in a variety of complaints such as diet induced constipation, giddiness, etc. A study by Thompson and Thomas in 1992 stated that most obese were likely to have negative views on their treatment by health professionals. Jennifer et. al. (2002) reported that women in distress consumed 118 kilocalories extra after enrolling in a weight-loss programme and social stress was found to be one of the main factors resulting into deviations. Emotional reasons such as boredom, stress and lack of family support have been identified as a major reason for eating.

OTHER METHODS LESS COMMONLY EMPLOYED

1. Psycho Therapy

It tells us to visualise food not as a commodity to be consumed subconsciously but to consciously consume the food and experience the resultant effect. For e.g.

1. Look at the bowlful of watermelon.
2. Think it to be a big serving that would satiate you.
3. Eat one piece at a time and chew it 10 times.
4. Wait before you take next piece.
5. By the time you have finished the bowl you feel satisfied.

Pat Yourself When You Succeed But Not With Food

Rewards that you can control can be used to encourage attainment of behavioural goals, especially those that have been difficult to reach. An effective reward is something that is desirable, timely, and contingent on meeting your goal. The rewards you administer may be tangible (e.g., a movie or music CD or a payment toward buying a more costly item) or intangible (e.g., an afternoon off from work or just an hour of quiet time away from family). Numerous small rewards, delivered for meeting smaller goals, are more effective than bigger rewards, requiring a long, difficult effort.

All dieters have bad days. So will you. Instead of relying on will power to guarantee continuous weight loss, plan ahead and how to cope. And remember, it is not the bad day that destroys your weight loss diet – it is the guilt you feel after bingeing that does the damage.

2. Drug Therapy

The most available weight loss medications are "appetite-suppressant" which promote weight loss by decreasing appetite by increasing serotonin or catecholamine or increasing the feeling of being full. Serotonin and catecholamine are the two brain chemicals which affect mood and appetite.

There are some chemicals in our brain that regulate food intake, energy expenditure and body weight. They control appetite by reducing hunger or increasing satiety. They may also increase total energy expenditure. These include:

1. Amphetamine like agents (e.g. Phentermine)
2. Phenylpropanolamine HCL
3. Fenfluramine
4. Sibutramine
5. Orlistat
6. Anti-diabetic agent (e.g. metformin)
7. Thyroid hormone
8. Recombinant human leptin
9. β-3 receptors

These drugs are not used frequently because of:
1. Side effects of these drugs
2. Rebound weight gain after stoppage of drug
3. Potential for drug abuse

Most of the medications approved are only for a short term use. Sibutramine and orlistat are the only drugs for weight loss which are approved for long term use in significant obese individual.

Side Effects of the Drugs

Most of the side effects of the medications are mild and improve as the condition improves. Some of the side effects of the drugs are as follows:

Medications affecting catecholamine levels: Symptoms of sleeplessness, nervousness, and feeling of well-being.

Sibutramine: Elevations in blood pressure and pulse. Hence people with heart pressure, high blood pressure, heart disease, irregular heart beats or history of stroke should not take this medication.

Orlistat: Oily spotting, gas with discharge, urgent need to go to bathroom, oily or fatty stools, increased number of bowel movements. These side effects are mild and temporary, but may become worse if high fat foods are eaten.

Orlistat reduces the absorption of some vitamins and hence patients should take multivitamin tablet.

Fenfluramine or Dexfenfluramine: Most of the patients who were taking fenfluramine or dexfenfluramine, either alone or in combination suffer from primary pulmonary hypertension (PPH) which is very rare but a disorder which affects the blood vessel in the lungs and results in death within four years.

Some Self-administered Methods of Weight Reduction and its Dangers

(a) Use of Ipecac Syrup
This syrup is used by individuals with eating disorders to induce vomiting. If used repeatedly it can weaken the heart muscle and cause chest pains, breathing problems, irregular heart beats and may lead to cardiac arrest and death.

(b) Use of Laxatives
Use of laxatives is perceived as a means to reduce weight by individuals with eating disorders. Although laxatives have little or no effect on reducing weight because by the time they work, the calories have already been absorbed. The person usually feels like they have lost weight because of the amount of fluid that is lost. That feeling is only temporary because the body will start to retain water within a 48 to 72-hour period. This usually leaves the person feeling bloated and induces him/her to fall into the vicious cycle of repeated use. Laxative abuse can cause bloody diarrhoea, electrolyte imbalances and dehydration. Prolonged use of laxatives can cause constipation, severe abdominal pain, nausea and vomiting and a permanent desire to bowels. Sometimes it may lead to severe medical complications and even death.

(c) Use of Diuretics (Water-Pills)
Diuretics do not cause weight loss, but repeated use can cause serious medical complications. When taken, a person will only lose vital fluids and electrolytes. Within a day or two the body will react and start to retain water, which is usually what causes a person to use them repeatedly. Abuse of diuretics usually leads to dehydration which can cause kidney damage. The use of diuretics for prolonged period cause electrolyte imbalances

that cause the failure of functioning of vital organs of the body such as heart, kidney and liver.

(d) Diet Pills
Refer drug therapy.

3. Surgery

This method is adopted in exceptional cases when the patient's BMI exceeds 40 kg/m² and when all the treatment methods have been failed. Such patients are at high risk for obesity-related morbidity and mortality. The surgery usually restricts the calorie intake (eg vertical banded gastroplasty) or combines the calorie restriction with some degree of malabsorption (eg biliopancreatic bypass)

With the surgery the patient can decrease a number of obesity related health complications like lowering of blood sugar levels, hypertension and the risk for heart disease.

Gastric Bypass Surgery

These surgeries can be classified into three types: restrictive, malabsorptive and a combination of restrictive and malabsorption.

The Roux-en Y is a restrictive type of surgery with minimal postoperative complications combined with a modified gastric bypass that works by decreasing food intake, limiting the amount of food, the stomach can hold by closing off a significant portion of the stomach and delaying the emptying of the stomach (gastric pouch).

Roux-en-y Gastric Bypass

In this operation the stomach is divided into two compartments with several rows of titanium staples. The newly-created stomach pouch is measured at less than 30 cc's. The small intestine is then divided in the proximal jejunum and the lower end brought up and joined to the new small stomach compartment. The pouch initially holds about 30 g of food and expands to 60 to 100 ml with time. The pouch's lower outlet usually has a diameter of about 1/2-inch. The small outlet delays the emptying of food from the pouch and causes a feeling of fullness. After an operation, the person usually can eat only 5 to 10 bites of food before feeling full. With time, the capacity may increase to half to a whole cup of food that may be consumed without discomfort or nausea. Food has to be well chewed. Some patients report that their tastes change after surgery. For most people, the ability to eat a large amount of food at one time is lost, but some patients do return to eating modest amounts of food without feeling hungry.

Many patients experience the "dumping syndrome" in which foods, usually those high in fat and/or sugar are not well tolerated. In the dumping syndrome stomach contents move too rapidly through the small intestine. Symptoms include nausea, weakness, sweating, faintness, and, occasionally, diarrhoea after eating these foods. Patients find that this negative incentive helps them to eliminate high caloric foods from their diets.

The postoperative risks include respiratory problems, infections, bleeding, bowel obstruction, leakage of the bowel connections, and obstruction of the stomach outlet. Gall bladder disease is a potential side effect due to the rapid weight loss most patients experience after the surgery. However appropriate medications may reduce its risk.

Contraindications for Surgery
There are some conditions that might disqualify you for surgery. Possible contraindications include alcoholism, hepatic cirrhosis with impaired liver functions, serious psychiatric disability, and correctable hormonal causes of obesity.

A morbidly obese individual can be considered for surgery after a medical evaluation which includes assessment of general fitness, blood tests, an ECG, a chest x-ray, a pulmonary function test, an upper gastrointestinal x-ray, a gall bladder ultrasound, and other tests as needed along with psychological screening. The purpose of the psychological screening is to ensure that there is no severe psychological issue that would compromise the chances for success on the programme, and to ensure that there will be adequate personalised support during the postoperative life.

Adequate nutritional counselling is also conducted to ensure appropriate dietary intake following the surgery.

4. Gastric Balloons and Jaw Wiring

In order to reduce the stomach capacity one of the techniques employed is introduction of gastric balloons in the stomach. The weight loss obtained with this method is low and there is a significant risk of gastric mucosal ulcers. Jaw wiring often results in weight loss as the patients food intake reduces. Such patients are able to take low calorie foods and many foods are restricted due to the loss of chewing capacity. Studies have shown that weight loss of about 36 kg could be achieved in 9 months with this technique. However this loss could not be sustained after the removal of the wires.

Counselling Techniques for Weight Loss

The counselling of the patients for obesity starts by collecting the history of the person. It can be collected using interview method to arrive at the treatment plan.

During the interviewing process care should be taken regarding complete attentiveness on the part of the counsellor and the environment should be free from interruptions. Psychological privacy and emotional objectivity should be given prime importance.

To identify the cause for obesity the personal history, dietary history and activity pattern of the person needs to be taken.

Personal history includes age, height, sex, weight, occupation of the person. Dietary history includes the consumption of the food items and activity pattern includes whether the person has sedentary, moderate or active lifestyle.

Measurement of complete body analysis is also important before starting a treatment. The Body Mass Index should be calculated, which tells in which grade of obesity the person belongs. Medical history should be taken by a physician to rule out any medical complications.

The factors that lead to obesity should be determined to arrive at an appropriate treatment plan. This should be followed by estimation of the possible weight loss by the individual.

For losing 1 kg of body weight one has to burn 7500 kcal. Suppose one is consuming 2000 cal/day and is still putting on weight, it means that she is not utilising all those calories and is stored in the form of fat. If the individual is advised to reduce the calorie intake to 1200 cal/day, there is reduction of 800 cal/day amounting to 5600 cal/week, and a brisk walk every day for 25 minutes will further make him/her to lose 100 cal/day, amounting to 700 cal/week. This will total upto 7600 cal/week, which is equivalent to losing 1 kg of fat. Any failure in adhering to the diet or exercise schedule will be reflected on the weighing scale.

After calculating the desirable weight loss per month, the diet for the person can be planned. The exchange list of the diet along with the sample menu should be handed to the patient (sample exchange list), advising to strictly follow the same.

The patient should also be advised to maintain a diet diary, recording when there was strong urge to eat food and what did he do as well as maintaining his daily diet and exercise. The patient then can be called for follow up after one month.

When the patient comes for the follow up, it should include the following:
1. Checking the weight loss.
2. Doing deviation analysis if desired weight loss is not achieved.
3. Counselling for the deviations.
4. Modifying the diet and exercise programme if necessary.

Are you Choosing a Correct Weight Loss Clinic?

If you choose to join a weight-reducing clinic make sure that the clinic is adhering to the golden rules of successful and sustained weight reduction.

1. Is the clinic run by trained and experienced dieticians?
2. Does the clinic promise a slow and steady weight reduction? Rapid weight loss is generally not sustained and results in weight cycling.
3. Does the diet plan include all the nutrients required by the body for each day except calories? Beware of the fad diets!!
4. Does the prescribed diet include severe restrictions? For e.g. a high protein diet with little or no carbohydrates.
5. Does the programme offer knowledge on long term weight maintenance and changes in the lifestyle pattern/ behaviour modification?
6. What is the success rate of the clinic in terms of individuals maintaining their reduced weight in the long run?

Children Imitate their Peers/Parents

A child's diet and his or her activity level both play an important role in determining whether that child will be underweight or overweight. The parents, must set an example. The popularity of television, the internet and video games all keep your child sitting around for hours doing nothing. An average Indian child spends more than four hours a day watching television, time that could be spent on creative activities for betterment of their future.

Such habits can run on generations and therefore it is necessary to stop it now.

If you think that your child is overweight now, it only gets worse, so at least discuss it with a diet consultant because hearing it from a professional sets them in motion to make positive change. Do not let anyone tell you that assessing obesity in children is difficult because children go through growth spurts. Fat is fat. We all know what it looks like.

These activities offer children hints about proper food preferences, teaching them about nutrition, and providing them with a feeling of intelligence.

Set a good example. Children are good learners, and they learn best by example. Setting a good example for your kids by eating a variety of good foods and being physically active yourself will teach your children lifestyle habits that they can follow and pass on to their families too.

Dealing with Your Toddlers' Eating Problems

It is common for toddlers to be picky. Their growth rate has slowed and their appetites may decrease. As they start to walk and run, they are often too busy to stop and eat. Many toddlers do not want to try new foods. All of this can be very frustrating for parents, but as long as your child's growth is good (ask your pediatrician), there is no need to worry.

Remember that you are responsible for planning, cooking, and serving nutritious meals and snacks at fairly regular times. This means three meals a day and, for toddlers, usually three snacks. Once you have put nutritious food on the table, let your child decide how much to eat and even whether or not to eat. Children will learn that if they are hungry, they have to find something to eat. Do not get in the habit of making special foods or giving little "handouts" throughout the day. Children will naturally eat enough to grow. They may only eat a fruit at lunch one day, but the next day they will make up for it by eating a chappati and vegetables.

Prevention of Obesity

Consumption of a balanced diet and moderate intensity activity is a sustainable way to maintain health and keep most of the diseases that are obesity related.

The following steps can be taken to prevent obesity:
1. Avoid excessive and frequent eating of foods rich in calories.
2. Take mild to moderate exercise daily.
3. Nutrition education to both mother and children will help to prevent obesity.
4. Prevention of obesity should start from infancy.

A group of 30 international experts commissioned by WHO has arrived at broad guidelines on what constitutes a healthy diet. These recommendations include:
  (a) Limiting fat to between 15 and 30 per cent of total daily energy intake.
  (b) Protein intake should be between 10 to 15 per cent of total calories.

(c) Saturated fats to less than 10%.

(d) Carbohydrates should provide the bulk of energy between 55 and 75 per cent of daily intake.

(e) Free sugars should remain below 10 per cent.

(f) Salt intake should be less than 5 grams a day and should be iodised.

(g) Intake of fruits and vegetables should be at least 400 grams.

Prevention of Obesity can Begin at Infancy

1. Plan and prepare healthy foods that are delicious and mouth-watering.
2. Plan weekly menu to include most of the food groups.
3. Frequent feeding should be avoided and let the child recognise true hunger and satiation.
4. Encourage children in the planning and preparing the meals.
5. Let mealtimes be a family event that involves participation of all members. A family that eats together stays together.
6. Limit the time spend on computers and television. Encourage more outside activities.
7. Do not shop for the foods that the children should not be eating.
8. Encourage consumption of soups and salads at the beginning of the meal when the children are really hungry and excess consumption of high calorie foods can be prevented.
9. Fast foods restaurants should be visited occasionally only on special events and not as a routine affair.

The overall goal of a successful treatment programme should be to help the whole family focus on making healthy changes to their eating and activity habits that they will be able to maintain throughout life and who better suited to do this than the family themselves.

1000 Calories Diet

Daily Menu Guide: The sample menu given below provides 1000 calories along with the various exchanges that can be selected from the exchange list given in the appendix no 1.

Exchange list for menu 1, 2 and 3

Items	Number of Exchanges	Amounts	Energy kcal	Protein gm	Fat gm
Milk and its products	2	500	145	16	–
Cereals	5	100	350	10	–
Pulses	1.5	45	150	10.5	–
Vegetable – A	3	300	–	–	–
Vegetable – B	2	200	80	4	–
Fruits	3	300	120	–	–
Fat	3	15	135	–	15
Sugar	1	5	20	–	–
		Total	1000	40.5	15

MENU 1

Breakfast	
Cereal: 1 exchange	Tea (50ml skimmed milk with 1 pill of sugar free): ½ cup
Fruits: 1 exchange	Skimmed milk with sugar free:
Milk: 1 exchange	1 glass
	Toast: 1 slice
	Papaya: ¾ cup
Lunch	
Cereal: 2 exchange	Mixed vegetable soup: 1 cup
Milk: 1 ½ exchange	Vegetables (blended) + pulse curry: 1 cup
Vegetable A: 2 exchange	Stuffed garden egg : ¾ cup
Vegetable B: 1.4 exchange	Chappaties (thin): 2 small
Pulses: 1 exchange	Mixed vegetable in curd: ¾ cup
Fat: 2 exchange	

Menu 1 contd...

Menu 1 contd...

Evening Fruits: 1.4 exchange Milk: ¼ exchange Sugar: ½ exchange	Tea: 1 cup Orange: One large
Dinner Cereal: 2 exchange Fruits: ½ exchange Milk: ½ exchange Vegetable A: 1 exchange Vegetable B: 0.6 exchange Pulses: ½ exchange Fat: 1 exchange Sugar: ½ exchange	Pulse soup: 1 cup Salad: 1 plate Lady's finger in curd: 1 cup Chappaties: 3 (sweet) Milk: ½ cup

MENU 2

Breakfast Cereal: 1 exchange Vegetable A: 1 exchange Milk: 1 exchange	Tea (50ml skimmed milk with 1 pill of sugar free): ½ cup Skimmed milk with sugar free: 1 glass Khakhra 2, small without oil
Lunch Cereal: 2 exchange Vegetable A: 2 exchange Vegetable B: 1 exchange Pulses: ½ exchange Fat: 1 exchange	Spinach soup: 1 cup Steamed bottle gourd: 1 cup Dal (thin): ¾ cup Chappaties (thin): 2 small Salad: 1 plate
Evening Fruits: 1 exchange	Fresh pineapple slices: 3 medium
Dinner Cereal: 2 exchange Fruits: 1 exchange Milk: 1 exchange Vegetable B: 1 exchange Pulses: 1 exchange Fat: 2 exchange Sugar: 1 exchange	Cooked Cauliflower: ½ cup Chappaties (Thin): 2 small Green gram dal: 1 cup Curd: ¼ cup Fruit custard (Skimmed milk with sugar free) (½ chickoo, ¼ banana and ¼ apple): 1 cup

MENU 3

Breakfast	
Cereal: 1 exchange Fruits: 1 exchange Milk: 1.2 exchange Sugar: 1 exchange	Tea (50ml skimmed milk with 1 pill of sugar free): ½ cup Skimmed milk with sugar free: 1 glass Puffed rice: 1 ½ cup Apple: 1 small
Lunch	
Cereal: 3 exchange Vegetable A: 1 exchange Vegetable B: 1 exchange Pulses: 5 exchange Fat: 1.5 exchange	Lady's finger vegetable: ½ cup Dal (thin): 1 cup Chappaties (thin): 2 small Salad: 1 plate Rice: ½ cup
Evening	
Pulses: 1 exchange Fruits: 1 exchange Fat: ½ exchange	Sprouts (green gram whole): ¾ cup Papaya: ¾ cup
Dinner	
Cereal: 1 exchange Fruits: 1 exchange Milk: 0.8 exchange Vegetable A: 2 exchange Vegetable B: 1 exchange Fat: 1 exchange	Vegetable pulao: 1 cup Spinach and tomato soup: 1 cup Curd: ¼ cup Fruit dish (Banana, pomegranate and chickoo): 1 cup

1200 Calories Diet

Daily Menu Guide: The sample menu given below provides 1200 calories along with the various exchanges that can be selected from the exchange list given in appendix no 1.

Exchange list for menu 1, 2 and 3

Items	Number of Exchanges	Amounts	Energy kcal	Protein gm	Fat gm
Milk and its products	2	500	145	16	-
Cereals	7	140	490	10.88	-
Pulses	2	60	200	12	-
Vegetable – A	3	300	-	-	-
Vegetable – B	2	200	80	-	-
Fruits	2	200	80	-	-
Fat	3	15	135	-	15
Sugar	3.5	17.5	70	-	-
		Total	1200	38.8	15

MENU 1

Breakfast Cereal: 1 exchange Fruits: 1 exchange Milk: 1 exchange Sugar: 2 exchange Vegetable A: 0.5 exchange Fat: 1 exchange	Tea (50ml skimmed milk with 1 pill of sugar free): 1 cup Skimmed milk with sugar free: 1 cup Upma: ½ *katori* Orange: 1 medium
Lunch Cereal: 3 exchange Vegetable A: 2.5 exchange Pulses: 1.3 exchange Fat: 1 exchange Milk: 0.5 exchange	Tomato soup: 1 cup Salad: 1 plate Chappati (thin): 3 small Rice: 1 tablespoon Palak: ½ cup Dal (medium thick): 1 cup
Evening Milk: ¼ exchange Sugar: 1.5 exchange Fruits: 1 exchange	Tea: 1 cup Banana: 1 small
Dinner Cereal: 3 exchange Pulses: 0.7 exchange Milk: 3/4 exchange Vegetable B: 2 exchange Fat: 1 exchange	Capsicum: ½ cup *Chole*: 2 tablespoon Chappati (medium): 2 small Curd: 1 cup Rice: 1 tablespoon

MENU 2

Breakfast	
Cereal: 2 exchange	Tea (50ml skimmed milk with 1 pill of sugar free): ¾ cup
Fruits: 1 exchange	
Milk: 1 exchange	*Bataka pauva*: 1 cup
Sugar: 1.5 exchange	Sweet lime: One medium
Vegetable B: 1 exchange	
Lunch	
Cereal: 3 exchange	Mixed vegetable: ¾ cup
Vegetable A: 1 exchange	Chappati (medium): 3
Vegetable B: 2 exchange	Vegetable salad: 1 plate
Pulses: 1 exchange	Dal (thin): 1 cup
Fat: 1 exchange	
Evening	
Milk: 1 exchange	Chickoo shake: 1 ½ cup
Sugar: 2 exchange	
Fruit: 1 exchange	
Dinner	
Cereal: 2 exchange	Chappati (medium): 1 cup
Pulses: 1 exchange	Lady's finger, vegetable: ½ cup
Vegetable B: 1 exchange	Dal (thin): 1 cup
Fat: 1 exchange	Rice: 2 tablespoon

7
Eating Disorders and Obstacles

1. Eating Disorders

Eating disorders include a range of conditions that involve an obsession with food, weight and appearance to an extent that a person's health and daily activities are adversely affected. These disorders are real, treatable medical illnesses that are characterised by irregular patterns of eating without the involvement of the conscious of the person.

Such disorders are characterised by extreme and unhealthy reduction of food intake or severe overeating accompanied by feeling of distress or extreme concern about body shape or weight. Researchers are investigating how and why initially voluntary behaviours, such as eating smaller or larger amounts of food than usual, at some point move beyond control in some people and develop into an eating disorder.

The risk factors known to predispose a person to eating disorder include sensitivity to changes in life especially separation from family, life stresses and inability to cope with them, sociocultural and genetic or any other trauma. Crash dieting for a prolonged period is a common factor precipitating eating disorders.

The eating disorders commonly encountered are anorexia nervosa, bulimia nervosa, binge eating and compulsive overeating. They affect people of all ages and sexes, though it is more widely spread amongst young women and men. However, the older men and women have also been falling a prey to such eating disorder as per the report of US DHHS Office on Women's Health, 2000.

This chapter will throw light on types of various eating disorders, their signs and symptoms and physical/medical complications.

Factors that Lead to Eating Disorders in Various Age Groups

The high incidence and prevalence of eating disorders especially anorexia nervosa and bulimia nervosa in the recent years and its treatment has become a challenging task for the dieticians, pediatricians, clinicians and psychiatrists.

It is common to see emaciated models on the cover page of the fashion magazines and on televisions. In fact, society is giving a wrong message of being thin as a requirement for success in the fashion industry. Unfortunately these models weigh nearly 23 per cent less than their ideal body weights that can be very dangerous. Teenagers need to realise that society's ideal body image is not achievable.

Eating less has become an obsession with the teenagers. They blindly follow fad diets and are deprived of adequate nutrition and ultimately become victims of various health problems including eating disorders.

During their childhood the girls are given to play with Barbie dolls that are extremely thin and beautiful. However, they are not explained that attaining this level of thinness is not practical and healthy in day-to-day life.

The diet and fashion industries are not totally to blame for society's passion with thinness. It is the people who demand diet books and products hoping that they may have some magical effect of making them thin and slim like the models. The society therefore needs to be educated in terms of creating awareness about the benefits of maintaining normal body weight, and that imitating the models can lead to serious health disorders. The long term success in life in terms of work efficiency at work place and home cannot be attained with poor health. Such attitudes may affect their job sustainability too.

It is becoming increasingly common to find young children falling a prey to eating disorders. There could be several factors responsible for this.

Sexual Abuse
It is observed that if children cannot control what is happening to their bodies during abuse they try to restrict their food intake or their weight.

Expression of Emotions
In homes where children are not allowed to express their feelings try to express their feelings indirectly by indulging in compulsive eating. Such indulgence helps them to overcome the feelings of fear, pain, sadness, loneliness, anger, etc.

Lack of Attention
In homes where the parents are involved with their own problems and are not able to pay attention to their children's difficulties the latter try to find comfort in food.

Parents Attitude Towards Food
Many children try to imitate their parents and adopt their eating behaviours. If the parents are preoccupied with their appearance and weight children will receive the message that looks are very important.

Gender Discrimination by Parents
In many families girls are given the message that being slim and thin will put her in a better position in matrimonial market, whereas boys are fed more so that they become big and strong. This gives a wrong message that may lead to eating disorders.

In case of adolescents the stresses of going through puberty may predispose an individual to eating disorders. They are becoming more independent and at the same time are highly influenced by their peer groups. For many, entering into puberty can be a very emotional, stressful, confusing, and frightening time. Many are unaware of the fact that the weight that is gained during this time is not permanent and desperately try to take the weight off which can lead them to some kind of eating disorders especially anorexia nervosa. They are exhilarated by the feeling of getting compliments by their peer group once they start losing weight. Going through puberty early can be very upsetting, especially if the teenager is being subjected to sexual advances. These advances can be so upsetting it may cause them to feel ashamed of their bodies, fear of becoming a woman like due to the weight gained during adolescent, they start indulging in starvation.

Other factors such as death of a close member in a family, the parents undergoing through a divorce and too caught up in their own lives and neglect the child, parents being too critical or alcoholic abuse may also lead to eating disorders in adolescents.

Management Strategies with Eating Disorders

It is important to teach our children to be proud of themselves. At the same time children need to know that they are being loved for what they are and not for what they look like. The value of healthy eating needs to be inculcated in them and they should be made aware that being thin is unhealthy.

It is important to spare time and talk to the child about what is bothering them so that instead of focusing on their food intake one can address to the real problems. One should never criticise the child and express shamefulness about his or her weight. Such an attempt will infact cause more feelings of self-hate and will lead the child to eat more for comfort.

Unhealthy habits towards food can develop if the child is forced to eat even if he or she does not wish to. Such behaviours on part of parents can cause a child to hate mealtimes.

Children should be encouraged to participate in physical activities instead of sedentary activities like watching TV or sitting on computers for long hours.

To troubleshoot the problems of eating disorder in adolescents schools should also take an active role by educating the students on the dangers of eating disorders and to help teach them that in order to succeed in life, their weight does not matter. Teachers and school counsellors should also be made aware of the signs to look for. If eating disorders are caught early, and the person is willing to accept the help that is available to them, the chances of recovery are greater.

Health and counselling services at all colleges need to make students aware that they can go to these places for help. They should provide the students with information to help educate them. They should also provide psychological, medical, and nutritional counselling. Many colleges do provide some of these services, but there are still many that need to start, especially for the students that are from out of town and do not have families to turn to for help. It would also be helpful for colleges to provide stress management classes for their students. Since there are such a high number of college students suffering with eating disorders, it would be helpful for the students to have a support group to attend. Being with others who know and understand how they feel can help to show them that they are not alone.

The more services that colleges provide for students suffering with eating disorders, the better their chances are for recovery and to learn to adjust and deal with all the pressures that go along with college life.

Eating disorders become a woman's way of escaping the daily pressures of life such as children becoming independent and leaving the family, infidelity on part of the husband and a false notion that the cause of infidelity is her gaining weight. Also other pressures of maintaining a perfect marriage, be a perfect mother, and have a perfect career leads to either gaining or losing weight.

Men do develop eating disorders including anorexia nervosa. However they do not frequently come forward with their problems. It is very difficult for men to reach out and ask for help because eating disorders are still supposed to be "women's disease". Men with eating disorders have low self-esteem, are perfectionists, over achievers, do not know how to express emotions, avoid conflict, put other's needs ahead of their own, feel unworthy and hate almost everything about themselves. Sometimes the problem is so severe that they avoid food that keeps them alive. Like women, men too enjoy getting compliments for their looks. They enjoy getting attention for losing weight and decide to keep losing.

2. Anorexia Nervosa

People who have anorexia nervosa develop unusual eating habits such as avoiding food and meals, picking out a few foods and eating them in small amounts, weighing their food, and counting the calories of everything they eat. Also, they may exercise excessively.

Most women and an increasing number of men are motivated by the strong desire to be thin and a fear of becoming obese. Anorexics consider themselves to be fat, no matter what their actual weight is. Often anorexics do not recognise they are underweight and may still "feel fat" at 35 kg. Anorexics close to death will show you on their bodies where they feel they need to lose weight. In their attempts to become even thinner, the anorexic will avoid food and taking in calories at all costs, which can result in death.

Typical Characteristics of Anorexic Persons

1. The anorexics are usually perfectionist.
2. They set very high standards for themselves and feel they always have to prove their competence.
3. Such people may also feel the only control they have in their lives is in the area of food and weight.
4. Their obsession for weight loss increases by each passing day and they always look forward to a decline in their weight on the weighing scales without bothering about getting into dangerous levels of body weight.
5. They usually block their feelings and emotions by focusing on calories and losing weight. For them, it is easier to diet then it is to deal with their problems directly.
6. The anorexics usually have low self-esteem and sometimes feel they do not deserve to eat.
7. The anorexics usually do not accept that anything is wrong with them.
8. Hunger is very strongly denied. They resist any treatment that could help them because the idea of therapy is seen only as a way to force them to eat.

Signs and Symptoms

(a) An intense and irrational fear of body fat and weight gain even when markedly underweight;

(b) Relentless determination to become thinner and thinner.

(c) A misperception of body weight and shape to the extent of feeling or seeing "fat" even when emaciated. Other symptoms include: becoming withdrawn, excessive exercise, fatigue, always being cold, muscle weakness, excuses for not eating meals (ie ate earlier, not feeling well), unusual eating habits (ie cutting food into tiny pieces, picking at food), noticeable discomfort around food, cooking for others, but not eating themselves, restricting food choices to only diet foods, guilt or shame about eating, depression, irritability, mood swings, evidence of vomiting, laxative abuse, diet pills or diuretics to control weight, irregular menstruation, amenorrhea (loss of menstruation), wearing baggy clothes to hide weight loss, frequently checking of weight on scale, headaches, fainting spells and dizziness, difficulty eating in public, very secretive about eating patterns, pale complexion (almost a pasty look) and no known physical illness that would explain weight loss.

Physical/Medical Complications
These include skin problems, dehydration, shortness of breath, irregular heartbeats, bloating, constipation, hair loss, stomach pains, decreased metabolic rate, edema (water retention), lanugo (fine downy hair), loss of bone mass, kidney and liver damage, electrolyte imbalances, osteoporosis, insomnia, anemias, cathartic colon (caused from laxative abuse), low potassium (most common cause of nocturnal cardiac arrest), cardiac arrest and death.

Duration of Condition
The course and outcome of anorexia nervosa vary across individuals: some fully recover after a single episode; some have a fluctuating pattern of weight gain and relapse; and others experience a chronically deteriorating course of illness over many years.

Treatment
Once they admit they have a problem and are willing to seek help, they can be treated effectively through a combination of psychological, nutritional and medical care.

The first goal for the treatment of anorexia is to ensure the person's physical health, which involves restoring a healthy weight (NIMH, 2002). Reaching this goal may require hospitalisation. Once a person's physical condition is stable, treatment usually involves individual psychotherapy and family therapy during which parents help their child to learn to eat again and maintain healthy eating habits on his or her own. Behavioural therapy also has been effective for helping a person return to healthy eating habits. Supportive group therapy may follow, and self-help groups within communities may provide ongoing support.

Early diagnosis and treatment increases the treatment's success rate. Use of psychotropic medication in people with anorexia should be considered only after weight gain has been established. Certain selective serotonin reuptake inhibitors (SSRIs) have been shown to be helpful for weight maintenance and for resolving mood and anxiety symptoms associated with anorexia.

The acute management of severe weight loss is usually provided in an inpatient hospital setting, where feeding plans address the person's medical and nutritional needs. In some cases, intravenous feeding is recommended. Once malnutrition has been corrected and weight gain has begun, psychotherapy (often cognitive-behavioural or interpersonal psychotherapy) can help people with anorexia, overcome low self-esteem and address distorted thought and behaviour patterns. Families are sometimes included in the therapeutic process.

Prognosis

An estimated 10 to 20% will eventually die from complications related to it. The mortality rate among people with anorexia has been estimated at 0.56 per cent per year, or approximately 5.6 per cent per decade, which is about 12 times higher than the annual death rate due to all causes of death among females in ages 15-24 years in the general population. The most common causes of death are complications of the disorder, such as cardiac arrest or electrolyte imbalance and suicide.

3. Bulimia Nervosa

Bulimia is eating large amounts of food secretly in a discrete period, in an automatic and helpless manner coupled with a sense of lack of control. Bulimia is characterised by self-perpetuating and self-defeating cycles of binge eating and purging. A person binges by rapidly consuming a large amount of food (or what she perceives to be a large amount). A binge is different for all individuals. For one person a binge may range from 1000 to 10,000 calories, for another, one cookie may be considered a binge. Purging methods usually involve vomiting and laxative abuse. Other forms of purging can involve excessive exercise, fasting, use of diuretics, diet pills and enemas.

Bulimics are usually people that do not feel secure about their own self-worth. They usually strive for the approval of others. They tend to do whatever they can to please others, while hiding their own feelings. Food becomes their only source of comfort. Bulimia also serves as a function for blocking or letting out feelings. Unlike anorexics, bulimics do realise they have a problem and are more likely to seek help.

Signs and Symptoms

These include binge eating and purging, secretive eating, feeling out of control while eating, frequent dieting, bathroom visits after eating, vomiting, laxative, diet pill or diuretic abuse, weight fluctuations (usually in 4-7 kg), belief that self-worth requires being thin, and extreme concern with body weight and shape, swollen glands, broken blood vessels, harsh exercise regimes, fasting, mood swings, depression, severe self-criticism, fear of not being able to stop eating voluntarily, self-deprecating thoughts following eating, fatigue and muscle weakness, tooth decay, irregular heartbeats, avoidance of restaurants, planned meals or social events, complains of sore throat, need for approval from others, substance abuse, including shoplifting or alcohol abuse, drugs, credit cards, sex etc.

Physical/Medical Complications

Most of the medical complications of bulimics resemble those of anorexics. However other complications include: tears of esophagus, erosion of teeth enamel, chronic sore throat, kidney and liver damage, parotid gland enlargement, low blood pressure, chest pains, development of peptic ulcers and pancreatitis (inflamation of the pancreas), gastric dilation and rupture abrasions on back of hands and knuckles.

Treatment

Unless malnutrition is severe, any substance abuse problem that may be present at the time of diagnosis is usually treated first. The next goal of treatment is to reduce or eliminate the person's binge eating and purging behaviour (NIMH, 2002). Behavioural therapy has proven effective in achieving this goal. Individual or group psychotherapy that uses cognitive-behavioural or interpersonal approach has proven effective in helping to prevent the eating disorder from recurring and in addressing issues that led to the disorder. Psychotropic medications, primarily antidepressants such as the selective serotonin reuptake inhibitors (SSRIs), have been found helpful for people with bulimia, particularly those with significant symptoms of depression or anxiety, or those who have not responded adequately to psychosocial treatment alone. These medications also may help prevent relapse.

It is helpful to establish a pattern of regular, non-binge meals, mechanisms to improve the attitudes related to the eating disorder, encouraging healthy and moderate exercise, and addressing the conditions such as mood or anxiety disorders are among the specific objectives of these strategies.

Prognosis

An estimated 1.1 per cent to 4.2 per cent of females have bulimia nervosa in their lifetime with symptoms such as at least two binge/purge cycles a week, on an average, for at least 3 months; lack of control over his or her eating behaviour; and seems obsessed with his or her body shape and weight (APA, 1994; NIMH, 2002) is normally observed.

4. Binge-eating Disorder

Binge-eating disorder is much like bulimia except the individuals do not use any form of purging (ie vomiting, laxatives, fasting, etc.) following a binge. Here the person is often genetically predisposed to weigh more than the "average" person. Individuals usually feel out of control during a binge episode, followed by feelings of guilt and shame.

The binge-eating episodes are associated with some of the following conditions i.e. they eat faster than the normal individuals until they feel too full for comfort, they tend to eat large quantities without any appetite arousal. They usually prefer to eat alone due to feeling of embarrassment of eating too much.

Signs and Symptoms

The signs and symptoms of binge eating are weight gain accompanied by fluctuations in weight, low self-esteem, depression and anxiety, loss of sexual desire, hiding food and secretive eating patterns, disgusted with self, going on many different diets, belief that life will be better if they lose weight, avoidance of social situations where food will be present, and suicidal thoughts.

Physical/Medical Complications

These include obesity, menstrual irregularities, diabetes, high blood pressure, high cholesterol, osteoarthritis, decreased mobility, shortness of breath, heart disease, liver and kidney problems, cardiac arrest and/or death.

Treatment

Like all eating disorders, binge eating is a serious problem but can be overcome through proper treatment. Diet programmes do not always work with patients of binge-eating disorder.

Eating disorders can be treated and a healthy weight restored. The sooner these disorders are diagnosed and treated, the better the outcomes are likely to be. Because of their complexity, eating disorders require a comprehensive treatment plan involving medical care and monitoring, psychosocial interventions, nutritional counselling and, when appropriate, medication management. At the time of diagnosis, the clinician must determine whether the person is in immediate danger and requires hospitalisation.

Diagnosis for Binge Eating

An individual who has at least two binge-eating episodes a week, on an average, for 6 months; and lacks control over his or her eating behaviour (NIMH, 2002) is said to be suffering from binge-eating disorder.

5. Compulsive Overeating

Compulsive overeating usually starts in early childhood when eating patterns are formed. It is characterised by uncontrollable eating and consequent weight gain. Most people who become compulsive eaters never learnt the proper way to deal with stressful situations and used food as means to cope with such conditions. They usually feel out of control and are aware that their eating patterns are abnormal. Like bulimics, compulsive overeaters do recognise they have a problem.

The individuals who have been victims of sexual abuse feel that being overweight will keep others at a distance and make them less attractive. Unlike anorexia and bulimia, there is a high proportion of male overeaters.

They usually undergo dieting to reduce weight but fall into the vicious circle of diet and binge eating. This is followed by feelings of powerlessness, guilt, shame and failure. Dieting and bingeing can go on forever if the emotional reasons for it are not dealt with.

In today's society, compulsive overeating is not yet taken seriously enough. Instead of being treated for the serious problem they have, they are instead directed to diet centres and health clinics. Like anorexia and bulimia, compulsive overeating is a serious problem and can result in death. With proper treatment, which should include therapy, medical and nutritional counselling, it can be overcome.

Signs and Symptoms

These are binge eating, fear of not being able to stop eating voluntarily, depression, self-deprecating thoughts following binges, withdrawing from activities because of embarrassment about weight, going on many different diets, eating little in public, while maintaining a high weight, believing they will be a better person when thin, feelings about self based on weight, social and professional failures attributed to weight, feeling tormented by eating habits, weight is focus of life.

Physical/Medical Complications

Weight gain, hypertension or fatigue, heart ailments, mobility problems, diabetes, arthritis, sciatica, varicose veins, hiatal hernia, embolism, sleep deprivation, toxemia during pregnancy, high blood pressure, shortness of breath, high cholesterol levels, cardiac arrest and death.

6. Night-eating Syndrome

Night-eating syndrome has not been formally defined as an eating disorder. It has its basis in the biological and emotional factors. Such a pattern persists for at least a period of 2 months where the individual feels tense, upset and guilty while eating. The major part of the food intake is usually taken after dinner and there is little or no appetite for breakfast. Such people find it difficult to sleep and untimely eating produces guilt and shame.

7. Nocturnal Sleep Related Eating Disorder

Nocturnal sleep-related eating disorder is not really an eating disorder but is thought to be a sleep disorder. Such incidence occurs when the person is somewhere between wakefulness and sleep, and may binge or consume strange combinations of food or non-food items. When awake, the person has little or no memory of the event.

8. Pica

Pica is usually found in individuals whose diets are deficient in minerals that are usually available from non-food items, such as dirt, clay, chalk, paint chips, cornstarch, baking soda, coffee grounds, cigarette ashes, rust, plastic, etc. There is a strong craving for these substances especially in pregnant women. Also people with psychiatric disturbances, or people whose family or ethnic customs include eating certain non-food substances are prone to such eating disorders. Pica is not always harmful unless substances are toxic or contaminated, and in this case can lead to medical emergency or death.

OBSTACLES IN LOSING WEIGHT

1. Weight Loss Plateau

The weight loss plateau can be described as a flattening out in the weight loss curve while following a diet or eating plan.

During this flattening of the curve weight loss ceases for a variable period of time. Many people become frustrated and believe that whatever eating plan they are following is not working. But such a belief is wrong. Because during this plateau phase the described changes in the liver and metabolism are happening even though it is not visible and such a phase is only temporary. Hence, one should continue to be impatient and revert back to eating but should carry out their modified diet and exercise.

2. Depression and Stress

Depression can lead to problems of increased body weight. This is because of the chemical imbalance existing within the brain of depressed people, that affects the appetite control centre in the brain.

Various methods to eradicate depression are as follows:
1. Joining a club with physical activities. Aqua aerobics can be the best exercise.
2. Having a regular therapeutic massage to relieve physical and emotional stresses.
3. Going for a walk each morning with a group of friends.
4. Seeking regular counselling from a psychotherapist or psychologist.
5. In case of severe depression physician may be consulted who may have put one on antidepressant medications.

3. Prevent Hypoglycemia and Trigger Foods

Hypoglycemia is a common cause of strong cravings for sweets and high GI carbohydrates. Once a person gets addicted or accustomed to eat high sugar foods, the body will expect them regularly and hence it is best to stop as soon as possible.

Some people need more chocolates and are chocolate addict. Although chocolate has a relative low GI but it is still high in fat and calories.

4. Lack of Exercise

Many people following a diet plan fail to maintain a regular exercise pattern. This can be due to busy time schedules, fatigue etc. But such practise should not be employed. Exercise should be done regularly.

Regular exercise will assist in increasing the metabolic rate and weight loss and thereby gradually improve the fitness levels.

5. Weight Cycling

Weight cycling is the repeated loss and regain of body weight. It is the result of dieting, often called "yo-yo" dieting.

The weight gain or loss can range from small weight change (2 – 5 kg/cycle) to large change (25 kg/cycle).

Some research links weight cycling with certain health risks. These include high blood pressure, high cholesterol, and gall bladder disease. To avoid potential risks, most experts recommend that irrespective of age, adopting of healthy eating and regular physical activity habits help to achieve and maintain a healthier weight for life.

A person who repeatedly loses and gains weight should not have more trouble trying to reach and maintain a healthy weight than a person attempting to lose weight for the first time.

Researchers have found that after a weight cycle, those who return to their original weights have the same amount of fat and lean tissue (muscle) as they did prior to weight cycling. People who exercise during a weight cycle may actually gain muscle.

Weight cycling can sometime have a negative psychological effect if you let yourself become discouraged or depressed.

8
Fad Diets and Myths

FAD DIETS

Fad diets are the ones that make individuals lose weight very quickly. But quick weight loss fools people because when they return to their normal diet they regain the lost weight immediately and sometimes gain double the weight that was lost. These fad diets can be hazardous to health.

Most of the fad diets are commonly known as crash diets. Some diets lead to losses in body fluids only and actually very little fat is lost. Some of the fad diets are as follows:

Such diets are not balanced in various nutrients, they are not realistic and difficult for people to follow on a long term basis.

1. The Atkins Diet

In the Atkins Diet, large amounts of fat and proteins are consumed whereas the carbohydrates are restricted, and thus the body will break down fat and muscle for energy.

But as large amount of fat is consumed it can increase the risk of heart disease. Moreover, increased breakdown of fat releases substances like ketones in the blood stream leading to ketosis.

These diets are generally considered low in carbohydrate and high in protein but usually are high in fat. The premise is that by avoiding carbohydrates, you will decrease your appetite. By avoiding some of the food groups (like vegetables), one can develop deficiencies of vitamins, especially vitamin A, the B group, C, and occasionally K. Additionally, since the diet is generally high in fat, serum lipids (cholesterol and triglycerides) tend to be higher. Rather than this a balanced calorie-deficit diet is safer and more likely to assist for a longer period of time.

2. The Hollywood Diet

In this diet a specially formulated combination of juices containing vitamins and minerals is consumed which claims to cleanse the body and promote weight loss. It is for a short term use and brings temporary results.

3. Grape Fruit Diet

This is based on an assumption that grapefruit has fat-burning enzymes and if taken before every meal, the calorie intake is restricted to 800 calories. But scientifically no such enzymes have still been found. In fact if this diet is taken then the person also drinks a large amount of caffeine.

4. Cabbage Soup Diet

Here only the cabbage soup is eaten for a week. But it does not provide the body all the nutrients and many people feel weak after a few days.

Such a diet severely lacks in calories.

5. A Three-Day Diet

There is a restricted calorie intake for three days (about 1000 cal) but after three days when shifted to normal diet, the weight lost regains quickly.

6. Fruits and Vegetables Diet

Fruits and vegetables are high in fiber, loaded with antioxidants and valuable phytochemicals, and can certainly provide fuel for energy. A fruit and vegetable based diet can lead an individual into a severe calorie deficiency. Since fruits are relatively low in calories compared to animal foods, nuts, dairy products, etc. Weight loss is usually attained, but it is short lived. Besides like any calorie restrictive diet, the fruits and vegetables diet leads to loss of lean body mass and water loss. The minimisation of complete proteins in random vegetarian diets often leads to further muscle catabolism (the body begins to feed off the muscle tissue for fuel) and over the time decline in energy metabolism. There are many vegetable based foods and food combinations including soy products, beans, whole grains, and nuts that can work together to fill in the amino acids and minerals that are most often delivered through meats and animal foods.

7. Myths and Realities

Myth: Getting attracted to commercial propaganda and believing that their products are the only solution for weight loss.

Reality: As of date there is no such product existing which can reduce the weight safely and miraculously. Such means of weight loss are neither scientific nor are they practical. One can lose weight quickly by using such products but quick weight loss is not recommended. A loss of only 2-3 kgs in a month is advisable which can be reduced after consultation with an experienced and qualified dietician.

Myth: Scale is an ideal indicator for weight loss progress.

Reality: Frequent use of scale (weekly) to judge the amount of weight loss may not necessarily depict the true picture of one's progress on a weight-reducing programme. The reduced weight on the scale may be indicative of either loss of water, muscle or fat. The loss of muscle may in reality reduce metabolic rate of the body and thereby reduce the rate of weight loss. Whereas the loss of water from the body will give a false belief of having lost fat. True picture can be obtained by using the scale once in a month or by getting a body composition analysis done.

Myth: The weight loss can be attained by using only a pill.

Reality: Pills promote weight loss by decreasing the appetite but it is not advisable. In addition to weight loss they also have different side effects. For e.g., drugs like sibutramine can cause elevations in blood pressure and pulse; fenfluramine or dexfenfluramine, either alone or in combination, may sometimes cause primary pulmonary hypertension (PPH) that may affect the blood vessel in the lungs and result in death within four years.

Myth: I cannot lose weight because I am on tours most of the time.

Reality: If you are eating out most of the time it is very important to have right knowledge on the caloric values of food items. Most of the menu provide a wide variety of food items to choose ranging from calorie dense foods to low calorie foods. It will therefore be wise to make the right choice that will help you to prevent gaining weight. For e.g. ordering for salad without dressing or selecting soups that are not cream based. Keeping a fast (missing one or two meals in a week and not substituting it with a high calorie item) once or twice a week helps.

Myth: I am over 50 and cannot exercise anymore.

Reality: Exercise does not necessarily mean walking briskly or swimming or cycling but activities raising the arms or lifting the legs can get one started and eventually get into an exercise programme and achieve the desired weight loss.

Myth: Although I am conscious about inclusion of low fat foods in my daily diet, I am not loosing weight.

Reality: You may be eating less fat and you may have reduced the percentage of calories that comes from fat in your diets, but your total calorie intake may be still higher than your total calorie output. To meet the dietary goals, you need to watch on your total calorie intake. The most effective way to keep lost weight off is to stay active. Always read the nutrition fact labels on the packets to judge your energy intake.

Myth: Low fat foods are tasteless.

Reality: Normal recipes of your choice can always be modified slightly to taste to your palate. Freshly prepared hot foods need not have lots of fat added to it. Use baked foods instead of deep fried foods. Use of fat substitutes to a small extent can enhance the palatability greatly.

Myth: Taking tea/coffee frequently does not add much to my calorie intake compared to fried foods

Reality: A calorie is a calorie whether it is coming from any of the food groups. What is important here is how much of that particular food is consumed. E.g. 4 cups of coffee a day (with 100 ml toned milk per cup) can contribute 440 calories compared to 216 calories coming from 20 pieces of potato chips.

Myth: Eating disorder is a problem of adolescents.

Reality: There is no age limit for the onset of eating disorders but even children and older men and women are known to be suffering from this.

Myth: It is impossible to completely recover from an eating disorder.

Reality: Although the duration of the treatment is long but consistent efforts on the part of caretakers and the team of doctors, dieticians and psychologists can help the individual to recover completely.

Myth: Anorexic persons can be easily judged by their appearance.

Reality: Many a times anorexic persons are weighing only about 5-10 kgs less than their normal weights and thus making it difficult for anybody to judge about the eating disorder they have.

Myth: Anorexics do not eat high calorie foods.

Reality: Most of the anorexics do avoid high calorie food but some are known to consume food items like chocolates, ice creams etc., substituting for the main meals of the day in such a way that their calorie intake per day does not increase beyond 300-500 kilo calories.

9
Approaches to Healthy Diet

The health of an individual is directly related to what he/she consumes in day-to-day life. Cooking habits need to be modified to balance the nutrients coming from the variety of food that one consumes.

Most of the Indian food preparations besides the routine *dal-chawal-roti-sabji* diet are calorie dense and if these preparations are consumed routinely as in many well to do families, it can lead to development of chronic degenerative disorders. Also, the Indian recipes provide a lot of scope for modification without substantially changing the physical and sensory qualities to suit to the need of the individuals with special requirements.

It was therefore attempted to develop standardised recipes that can be used in various therapeutic conditions by modifying their compositions. These include the recipes that are protein rich, low sugar sweets, high in fibre, iron rich, calcium rich and low calorie foods. Along with the ingredients and the steps to prepare these products, detailed nutritive values for these recipes are also given.

1. PROTEIN RICH RECIPES

PUNA MISAL

Ingredients

Green gram, whole	- 20 gm
Bengal gram, whole	- 20 gm
Rice flakes	- 15 gm
Curd	- 40 gm
Sugar	- 15 gm
Onion, chopped	- 15 gm
Tomato, chopped	- 15 gm

For Chutney

Coriander, whole	- 15 gm
Green chilli	- 5 gm
Tamarind	- 15 gm
Jaggery	- 10 gm
Salt	- to taste
Cumin powder, roasted	- ½ tsp

Preparation Steps

- Sprout green gram and Bengal gram.
- To prepare chutney, soak tamarind and jaggery for an hour and then grind them. Add salt, chilli powder and roasted cumin powder to it.
- Sweeten curd by adding sugar to it.
- Soak rice flakes for 5 mins.
- Finally, mix the sprouted green gram, Bengal gram, soaked rice flakes (for 5 mins), sweet curd, chutney, onion and tomato.

Nutritive Value

Calories	- 328	kcal
Protein	- 11.27	gm
Fat	- 3.17	gm
Iron	- 7.9	mg
Calcium	- 176.83	mg
Phosphorous	- 231.65	mg
Fibre	- 2.75	gm
Vitamin C	- 6.75	mg

DAL VADA

Ingredients

Bengal gram	- 50 gm
Ginger	- 5 gm
Garlic	- 3-4 flakes
Green chillies	- 2 (medium)
Salt	- to taste
Oil for frying	- 10 ml

Preparation Steps

- Soak Bengal gram for 2 hours.
- Semi-grind it in a mixer. Remove and transfer to a bowl.
- Add crushed ginger, garlic, green chillies and salt to it.
- Shape into rounds Deep fry in the pan and serve it with chopped onions.

Nutritive Value

Calories	- 288	kcal
Proteins	- 10.4	gm
Fats	- 12.10	gm
Iron	- 3.10	mg
Calcium	- 32.0	mg
Phosphorous	- 165.5	mg
Fibre	- 1.1	gm
Vitamin C	- 7.0	mg
B-Carotene	- 75.25	µg

Egg Sandwich

Ingredients

Eggs	- 60 gm
Butter	- 10 gm
Onion, chopped	- 15 gm
Green chillies, chopped	- 1 medium
Salt	- to taste
Bread	- 50 gm (2 slices)
Capsicum, chopped	- 10 gm
Red chilli powder	- to taste

Preparation Steps

- Beat the eggs.
- Add chopped onion, capsicum, green chillies, salt and red chilli powder.
- Heat butter in a pan.
- Pour the batter and spread around and then shallow fry.
- Cut it into small pieces and put it in between the two slices for making a sandwich.
- Grill in a sandwich maker.

Nutritive Value

Calories	- 366	kcal
Proteins	- 16.32	gm
Fats	- 20.47	gm
Iron	- 2.45	mg
Calcium	- 67.1	mg
Phosphorous	- 211.6	mg
Fibre	- 0.69	gm
Vitamin C	- 16.2	mg
B-Carotene	- 522.45	µg

Moong Dal Thepla

Ingredients

Green gram flour	- 50 gm
Curd	- 5 gm
Oil	- 5 gm
Ginger	- 5 gm
Green chillies	- 2
Cumin seeds	- ½ tsp
Salt	- to taste
Water	- 20 ml
Oil for shallow frying	- 10 ml

Preparation Steps

- Put green gram flour in a bowl and pour oil.
- Add curd, ginger, crushed green chillies, cumin seeds and salt.
- Make a dough with water and keep it for ½ to 1 hour to make it soft while applying.
- Divide the dough into small portions and roll them.
- Roast on a pan using oil.

Nutritive Value

Calories	- 316	kcal
Proteins	- 12.15	gm
Fats	- 15.85	gm
Iron	- 2.21	mg
Calcium	- 47.0	mg
Phosphorous	- 211.7	mg
Fibre	- 0.65	gm
Vitamin C	- 2.57	mg
B-carotene	- 31.55	µg

Approaches to Healthy Diet • 111

Lilwa Paratha

Ingredients

For Filler

Red gram, tender	- 50 gm
Oil	- 5 ml
Sugar	- 10 gm
Cumin seeds	- a pinch
Green chillies, chopped	- 2 number
Coriander leaves	- 5 gm
Gingelly seeds	- ½ tsp
Oil for shallow frying	- 5 ml
Salt	- to taste

For Dough

Wheat flour	- 25 gm
Oil	- 3 ml
Water	- 10 ml

Preparation Steps

For Filler

- Pour oil into a pan and add cumin seeds.
- Add crushed red gram tender, chopped green chillies, sugar, gingelly seeds, salt and coriander leaves.
- Sauté it and let it simmer.
- Mix properly and allow it cool.

For Dough

- Take wheat flour and pour oil and add salt to it.
- Make dough with water.
- Divide it into small equal portions.
- Roll the dough and fill with the filler. Close the seam properly and roll it again.
- Shallow fry adding oil on a pan.

Nutritive Value

Calories	- 303	kcal
Proteins	- 8	gm
Fats	- 14.0	gm
Iron	- 2.71	mg
Calcium	- 52.4	mg
Phosphorous	- 170.85	mg
Fibre	- 3.62	gm
Vitamin C	- 24.8	mg
B-carotene	- 596.4	µg

2. LOW SUGAR SWEETS

Vedmi

Ingredients

For Filler

Red gram dal	- 30 gm
Sugar	- 5 gm
Sweetner	- 1 pill of *equal* (artificial sweetner)
Cardamom powder	- a pinch
Poppy seeds	- a pinch
Water	- 30 ml
Ghee	- 5 ml

For Dough

Wheat flour	- 25 gm
Oil	- 3 ml
Water	- 10 ml

Preparation Steps

For Filler
- Pressure cook red gram dal till it becomes thick in consistency.
- Add sugar and sweetner.
- Then add cardamom powder and poppy seeds.
- Let it cool.

For Dough
- Add oil to wheat flour. Mix well.
- Make dough by adding water.
- Divide the dough into equal portions.

For Vedmi
- Roll the dough, fill the filler and close the seam properly.
- Then roll it again and shallow fry in a pan and apply ghee.

Nutritive Value

Calories	-	278	kcal
Proteins	-	9.71	gm
Fats	-	8.93	gm
Iron	-	2.03	mg
Calcium	-	34.5	mg
Phosphorous	-	180	mg
Fibre	-	0.92	gm
Vitamin C	-	0	mg
B-carotene	-	77	µg

BASUNDI

Ingredients

Milk	-	350 ml
Sugar	-	5 gm
Sweetner	-	1 pill of *equal*

Preparation Steps

- Boil milk till the volume reduces to half the original quantity. Stir in between.
- Add sugar and sweetner.
- Cook for a few more minutes and then let it cool.
- Garnish it with almonds and pistachios.

Nutritive Value

Calories	-	429	kcal
Proteins	-	15.0	gm
Fats	-	23	gm
Iron	-	0.7	mg
Calcium	-	736	mg
Phosphorous	-	455.05	mg
Fibre	-	0	gm
Vitamin C	-	3.5	mg
B-carotene	-	168	µg

KHAJUR PAK

Ingredients

Fresh dates	-	25 gm (seedless)
Khoa	-	20 gm
Ghee	-	10 gm

Preparation Steps

- Heat ghee in a pan.
- Add seedless fresh dates and khoa.
- Sauté till it is cooked.
- Smash it into a homogeneous mass.
- Let the ghee separate. Allow to cool.
- Make small equal balls of it.
- Garnish it with coconut powder.

Nutritive Value

Calories	- 210	kcal
Proteins	- 3.22	gm
Fats	- 16.34	gm
Iron	- 1.4	mg
Calcium	- 135.5	mg
Phosphorous	- 93.7	mg
Fibre	- 0.92	gm
Vitamin C	- 1.2	mg
B-carotene	- 27	µg

Sheera

Ingredients

Semolina	-	25 gm
Milk	-	50 ml
Ghee	-	10 gm
Sugar	-	05 gm
Sweetner	-	1 pill of *equal*
Cardamom powder	-	a pinch

Preparation Steps

- Heat ghee in a pan.
- Add semolina and sauté.
- Add milk, sugar and sweetner and boil till the ghee separates out and stir between boiling.
- Then add cardamom powder.
- Garnish with almond and piyal seeds.

Nutritive Value

Calories	- 255	kcal
Proteins	- 4.75	gm
Fats	- 13.45	gm
Iron	- 0.5	mg
Calcium	- 109.6	mg
Phosphorous	- 90.55	mg
Fibre	- 0.05	gm
Vitamin C	- 0.5	mg
B-carotene	- 84	µg

Dudhi Halwa

Ingredients

Bottle gourd	-	40 gm
Sugar	-	05 gm
Ghee	-	08 gm
Sweetner	-	1 pill of *equal*
Khoa	-	10 gm
Milk	-	20 ml

Preparation Steps

- Heat ghee in a pan.
- Add grated bottle gourd along with *khoa*.
- Add milk and stir so it becomes homogenous.
- Add sugar and sweetner.
- Sauté till the ghee separates.
- Let it cool and garnish it with almonds and cashewnuts.
- Make small equal pieces.

Nutritive Value

Calories	- 140	kcal
Proteins	- 2.40	gm
Fats	- 12.46	gm
Iron	- 0.49	mg
Calcium	- 149.6	mg
Phosphorous	- 95.05	mg
Fibre	- 0.24	gm
Vitamin C	- 0.8	mg
B-carotene	- 54.2	µg

3. LOW FAT RECIPES

Muthia and Chutney

Serving size: 1 medium serving

Ingredients: (Muthia)

Wheat flour (coarse)	- 70 gm
Bottle gourd	- 40 gm
Oil	- 03 ml
Sugar	- 05 gm
Garlic	- 1-2 flakes, grated
Turmeric powder	- ½ teaspoon
Red chilli powder	- 1 teaspoon
Salt	- to taste
Soda	- a pinch

Ingredients: (Chutney)

Coriander leaves	- 30 gm
Lemon juice	- 1 tablespoon
Salt	- to taste
Green chilli	- 1-2

Preparation Steps: (Muthia)

- Peel bottle gourd and grate it.
- Add wheat flour, grated garlic, salt, turmeric, red chilli powder into the grated bottle gourd and mix all the ingredients.
- Add water and make a dough of it.
- Make rolls and steam them for 10-15 minutes.
- Remove the rolls and cut them into small pieces.
- Shallow fry in oil by adding mustard seeds in it.
- Serve it with green chutney.

Preparation Steps: (Chutney)

- Wash coriander leaves and cut it.
- Add 1-2 chillies, lemon juice and salt in it.
- Blend in a blender and serve.

Nutritive Value

Calories	-	321	kcal
Proteins	-	9.54	gm
Fats	-	4.41	gm
Iron	-	4.04	mg
Calcium	-	80.66	mg
Phosphorous	-	295	mg
Fibre	-	2.56	gm
Vitamin-C	-	52.5	mg
B-carotene	-	2114.60	µg

Methi Debhra

Serving size: one.

Ingredients

Wheat flour	- 50 gm
Sugar	- 10 gm
Oil	- 5 ml
Fenugreek leaves	- 50 gm
Coriander powder	- ½ tsp
Turmeric powder	- ½ tsp
Garlic	- 2 cloves of garlic
Salt	- to taste

Preparation Steps

- Take wheat flour and add fenugreek leaves, sugar, salt, coriander powder, turmeric and garlic in it.
- Make dough with water.

- ➤ Divide into three portions and shape into balls. Shallow fry it.
- ➤ Serve hot with green chutney.

Nutritive Value

Calories	-	287.71 kcal
Proteins	-	8.57 gm
Fats	-	6.10 gm
Iron	-	4.35 mg
Calcium	-	224.2 mg
Phosphorous	-	203.72 mg
Fibre	-	1.56 gm
Vitamin-C	-	26.65 mg
B-carotene	-	1184.5 µg

WHOLE WHEAT GHUNGRI (NAMKEEN)

Serving size: one.

Ingredients

Whole wheat	- 50 gm
Tomato	- 50 gm
Oil	- 5 ml
Salt	- to taste
Red chilli powder	- to taste
Water	- 100 ml
Onion	- 25 gm

Preparation Steps

- ➤ Soak wheat overnight.
- ➤ Add water and cook it in a pressure cooker for 5 minutes.
- ➤ Chop onions and tomatoes.
- ➤ Heat oil in a pan.
- ➤ Add chopped onions and fry till it turns slightly brown in colour.
- ➤ Add chopped tomatoes to it.
- ➤ Add red chilli powder and salt and mix well.
- ➤ Mix with cooked wheat.
- ➤ Serve hot.

Nutritive Value

Calories	-	243 kcal
Proteins	-	6.80 gm
Fats	-	5.87 gm
Iron	-	3.27 mg
Calcium	-	54.40 mg
Phosphorous	-	178.50 mg
Fibre	-	1.15 gm
Vitamin-c	-	14 mg
B-carotene	-	211 µg

WHOLE WHEAT GHUNGRI (SWEET)

Serving size: one.

Ingredients

Whole wheat	- 50 gm
Jaggery	- 20 gm
Ghee	- 05 ml
Water	- 100 ml

Preparation Steps

- ➤ Soak wheat overnight.
- ➤ Add water and cook in a pressure cooker for 5 minutes.
- ➤ Add ghee and jaggery and mix well.
- ➤ Serve hot.

Nutritive Value

Calories	-	295 kcal
Proteins	-	5.98 gm
Fat	-	5.77 gm
Iron	-	3.17 mg
Calcium	-	36.50 mg
Phosphorous	-	161 mg
Fibre	-	0.60 gm
Vitamin-c	-	0 mg
B-carotene	-	45.5 µg

Idla and Coriander Chutney

Serving size: one.

Ingredients: (Idla)

Black gram dal	-	209 gm
Rice raw, milled	-	50 gm
Salt	-	to taste
Green chillies	-	3 in number
Water	-	50 ml
Oil	-	50 gm
Black pepper (dry)	-	a pinch

Ingredients: (Chutney)

Coriander leaves	-	25 gm
Ginger	-	2.5 gm
Green chillies		-1-2 in number
Salt	-	to taste

Preparation Steps

For Idla

- Mix black gram dal and rice in water and keep it for 7 to 8 hours.
- Then blend and allow it to ferment by keeping it for 7-8 hours again.
- Then add salt to the fermented product and little water so that the consistency is spreadable.
- Fill the water in the Idla cooker.
- Greeze the Idla dish with oil.
- Pour the fermented product in the dish and keep the dish in the cooker and sprinkle black pepper (dry) on it.
- Steam for 10 minutes or till it becomes soft.
- Take out the dish and cut it into equal size pieces.

For Chutney

- Wash coriander leaves and cut it.
- Add green chillies, ginger and salt to it.
- Blend it.

Nutritive Value

Calories	-	283.56 kcal
Proteins	-	12.23 gm
Fat	-	5.58 gm
Iron	-	2.96 mg
Calcium	-	77.45 mg
Phosphorous	-	158.18 mg
Fibre	-	1.01 gm
Vitamin-C	-	16.8 mg
B-carotene	-	452.4 µg

Dhudhpak

Serving size: 200 ml (1 cup)

Ingredients

Skimmed milk	- 600 ml
Rice	- 10 gm
Sugar	- 5 gm
Piyal seeds	- 1 tsp
Cardamom	- 1 gm

Preparation Steps

- Boil the milk for 5 minutes.
- Then add rice in it.
- Allow it to boil again till it becomes a little thick in consistency.
- Then add sugar in it and mix it properly.
- When it cools garnish with piyal seeds and cardamom.

Nutritive Value

Calories	-	263.49	kcal
Proteins	-	16.94	gm
Fats	-	3.62	gm
Iron	-	2.34	mg
Calcium	-	736.26	mg
Fibre	-	0.41	gm
Vitamin-c	-	0.25	mg
B-carotene	-	0	µg
Phosphorus	-	584.05	mg

BESAN DHOKLA

Ingredients

Bengal gram, whole	-	40 gm
Fenugreek leaves	-	20 gm
Turmeric powder	-	to taste
Red chilli powder	-	to taste
Coriander leaves	-	10 gm
Lemon juice	-	5 ml
Mustard seeds	-	Pinch
Niger seeds	-	Pinch
Water	-	1 cup

Preparation Steps

➤ Add 1 cup water in Bengal gram (*besan*).
➤ Add all the spices.
➤ Cook it on a medium flame till it forms a paste.
➤ Add fenugreek leaves.
➤ Spread it in a greezed plate.
➤ Let it cool.
➤ Cut it into desired pieces.
➤ Boil oil, mustard seeds and niger seeds separately and then spread it on the pieces.

Nutritive Value

Calories	-	166	kcal
Proteins	-	8.1	gm
Fats	-	2.40	mg
Iron	-	2.23	mg
Calcium	-	181.7	mg
Phosphorous	-	142.6	mg
Fibre	-	1.98	mg
Vitamin-C	-	1.99	mg
B-carotene	-	1235.4	µg

CHANA CHAT

Ingredients

Chickpeas	-	20 gm
Butter	-	3 gm
Tomatoes	-	20 gm
Onions	-	20 gm
Salt	-	to taste
Turmeric powder	-	a pinch
Red chilli powder	-	a pinch
Garam masala	-	a pinch
Coriander leaves	-	2-3 gm

Preparation Steps

➤ Soak chickpeas for 4 hours.
➤ Pressure cook it for 10 minutes.
➤ Heat the butter and sauté chopped onions and tomatoes in it.
➤ Add all the spices.
➤ Garnish it with coriander leaves.
➤ Serve warm.

Nutritive Value

Calories	-	57.59	kcal
Proteins	-	2.07	gm
Fats	-	2.53	gm

Iron	-	0.712	mg
Calcium	-	27.12	mg
Phosphorous	-	45.93	mg
Fibre	-	1.18	gm
Vitamin-C	-	11.65	mg
B-carotene	-	326.14	µg

Vegetable Soup

Ingredients

Cornflour	-	10 gm
Cauliflower	-	20 gm
Cabbage	-	15 gm
Carrot	-	10 gm
Peas	-	10 gm
Oil	-	01 ml
Green chillies, crushed	-	1-2
Ginger	-	to taste
Water	-	1½ cup
Milk	-	10 ml

Preparation Steps

➤ Pour oil into a pan.
➤ Add crushed green chillies and ginger paste.
➤ Add all the vegetables.
➤ Cook it for 5 minutes.
➤ Add water and let it boil for 10 minutes.
➤ Add cornflour.
➤ Add milk and serve.

Nutritive Value

Calories	-	45.65	kcal
Proteins	-	2.07	gm
Fats	-	1.21	gm
Iron	-	0.72	mg
Calcium	-	23.35	mg
Phosphorous	-	97	mg
Fibre	-	1.1	gm
Vitamin-C	-	31.6	mg
B-carotene	-	253.3	µg

4. HIGH FIBRE CUISINE

Niger Seeds Chikki

Ingredients

Niger seeds	-	110 gm
Gingelly seeds	-	50 gm
Jaggery	-	100 gm

Preparation Steps

➤ Take jaggery in a pan and add little water so that it melts and mixes properly till the jaggery becomes hot.
➤ Then add niger seeds and gingelly seeds and mix it. Then immediately switch off the flame.
➤ Take the mixture and pour on a clean flat surface. Roll it and cut it into pieces.
➤ Serve.

Nutritive Value

Calories	-	1231	kcal
Proteins	-	35.84	gm
Fats	-	64.65	gm
Iron	-	69.66	mg
Calcium	-	1135	mg
Fibre	-	13.44	gm
Vitamin-C	-	30	mg
B-carotene	-	—	µg

Shirkhoorma

Serving size: 250 ml

Ingredients

Coconut dry	-	151.5	gm
Skimmed milk	-	500	ml
Sugar	-	25	gm
Cardamoms	-	1	gm
Almonds	-	2	gm
Cashewnuts	-	2	gm

Preparation Steps

- Grind half coconut so that it becomes liquid like.
- Take the other half and roast in a pan for 5 minutes.
- Then add liquid coconut and skimmed milk. Boil it for 10 minutes.
- Add sugar in it and mix for 2 minutes.
- Add almond, cardamom and cashewnut in powder form.
- Serve.

Nutritive Value

Calories	-	1264.81	kcal
Proteins	-	23.67	gm
Fats	-	96.088	gm
Iron	-	12.99	mg
Calcium	-	1209.9	mg
Fibre	-	10.16	gm
Vitamin-C	-	15.5	mg
B-carotene	-	1.2	µg

Kachori and Tomato Chutney

Serving size: six.

Ingredients: (Kachori)

Red gram, tender	- 125 gm
Wheat flour, refined	- 600 gm
Coriander	- 5 gm
Salt	- to taste
Red chilli powder	- to taste
Turmeric powder	- to taste
Ginger	- 5 gm
Chillies	- 2 in number
Garam masala	- a pinch
Lemon juice	- 5 ml
Sugar	- 1 tsp
Oil	- 20 ml

Ingredients: (Tomato Chutney)

Tomatoes	- 100 gm
Salt	- to taste
Black pepper	- a pinch

Preparation Steps: (Kachori)

For Filler

- Crush red gram tender in a grinder.
- Crush ginger and green chillies separately.
- Stir it well for 5-10 minutes.
- Add salt, red chilli powder, turmeric powder, garam masala and stir it well till it becomes homogeneous.
- Add crushed ginger and green chillies in it.
- In the end add lemon juice and sugar.

For Dough
- Take wheat flour and pour 5 ml oil into it.
- Make a dough with water.
- Divide it into equal pieces and roll it into puris.
- Fill the prepared filler in the centre of the puri.
- Close all the four sides of the puri in such a way that it does not open.
- Pour oil in a frying pan and fry one by one.
- Serve hot.

For Tomato Chutney
- Cut tomatoes into small pieces.
- Boil it in its own juice till it becomes thick.
- Then at the end add salt and black pepper.
- The tomato chutney is ready to be eaten.

Nutritive Value

Calories	- 489.85	kcal
Proteins	- 19.93	gm
Fats	- 24.0	gm
Iron	- 3.67	gm
Calcium	- 195	mg
Phosphorous	- 298	mg
Fibre	- 8.7	gm
Vitamin-C	- 56.37	mg
B-carotene	-1128	µg

POMEGRANATE JUICE

Ingredients

Pomegranate	- 250 gm
Sugar	- 10 gm
Water	- 1 tablespoon

Preparation Steps
- Take cleaned pomegranate.
- Crush it in a mixer in thick form.
- Crush all the seeds properly.
- Add desired amount with water and sugar.

Nutritive Value

Calories	- 202.3	kcal
Proteins	- 4.01	gm
Fats	- 0.25	gm
Iron	- 4.48	mg
Calcium	- 26.2	mg
Phosphorous	- 175.1	mg
Fibre	- 12.75	gm
Vitamin-C	- 40	mg
B-carotene	- 0	µg

5. IRON RICH FOODS

CHANA CHAT

Serving Size: 1

Ingredient

Bengal gram	- 50 gm
Onion	- 25 gm
Tomato	- 25 gm
Oil	- 2.5 gm
Salt	- to taste
Red chilli powder	- to taste
Lemon juice	- to taste
Chat masala	- to taste

Preparation Steps

- Soak Bengal gram whole overnight.
- Cook in a pressure cooker and drain.
- Finely chop tomatoes and onion.
- Finally add chopped tomatoes, onion to the roasted Bengal gram and pour lemon juice over it.
- Add salt, red chilli powder and chat masala as per taste.
- Serve with *kathi methi* chutney. It can also be served with fresh curd and cumin seed powder.

Nutritive Value

Calories	-	228.25 kcal
Proteins	-	11.075 gm
Fats	-	5.315 gm
Iron	-	3.11 mg
Calcium	-	50 mg
Phosphorous	-	85.5 mg
Fibre	-	0.95 gm
Vitamin-C	-	7.75 mg
B-carotene	-	156 µg

PATRA

Serving size: 1 cup = 162 gm

Ingredients

Gram flour	-	50 gm
Sesame seeds	-	2.5 gm
Colocasia leaves	-	50 gm
Oil	-	05 ml
Turmeric powder	-	to taste
Salt	-	to taste
Red chilli powder	-	to taste

Preparation Steps

- Mix gram flour, salt, red chilli powder and turmeric powder with enough water to make a batter of dropping consistency.
- Apply the batter as a fine layer on colocasia leaves.
- Shape the leaf into a long roll.
- Steam the roll for 10 to 15 minutes and then cut it into thin slices.
- Season it with the gingelly seeds.
- Serve hot.

Nutritive Value

Calories	-	273.07 kcal
Proteins	-	12.8 gm
Fats	-	9.63 gm
Iron	-	7.88 mg
Calcium	-	177.75 mg
Phosphorous	-	220.75 mg
Fibre	-	2.12 gm
Vitamin-C	-	6.5 mg
B-carotene	-	5202 µg

PLAINTAIN BHAJIYA

Serving size: 12 numbers

Ingredients

Plaintain green	-	100 gm
Gram flour	-	50 gm
Oil	-	20 ml
Salt	-	to taste
Red chilli powder	-	to taste
Aniseed	-	to taste
Turmeric powder	-	to taste
Ginger-garlic paste	-	to taste

Preparation Steps

- Cut plaintain into thin slices.
- Mix the gram flour, salt, red chilli powder, cumin powder, aniseed, turmeric powder, ginger-garlic paste and a pinch of soda with enough water to make a batter of dropping consistency.
- Dip the plaintain slices in the batter and deep fry in hot oil until golden brown.
- Serve hot with tomato ketchup.

Nutritive Value

Calories	- 430	kcal
Proteins	- 11.8	gm
Fat	- 23	gm
Iron	- 8.92	mg
Calcium	- 38	mg
Phosphorous	- 194.5	mg
Fibre	- 1.3	gm
Vitamin-C	- 24.5	mg
B-carotene	- 94.5	μg

RAISINS-DATES SHAKE

Serving size: 75 gm

Ingredients

Dates	- 50 gm
Raisins	- 25 gm
Milk	- 200 ml

Preparation Steps

- Wash dates and remove seeds overnight.
- Soak the dates and raisins in milk. Refrigerate.
- Blend the contents in a liquidiser.
- Serve chilled.

Nutritive Value

Calories	- 383	kcal
Proteins	- 9.65	gm
Fats	- 13.27	gm
Iron	- 2.8	mg
Calcium	- 452.75	mg
Phosphorous	- 299	mg
Fibre	- 2.125	mg
Vitamin-C	- 2.25	mg
B-carotene	- 96.6	μg

PULSE SANDWICH

Serving size: 200 gm

Ingredients

Bengal gram, whole	- 25 gm
Green gram, whole	- 25 gm
Bread (2 slices)	- 30 gm
Mango powder	- 1/4
Salt	- to taste
Red chilli powder	- to taste
Cumin powder	- a pinch

Preparation Steps

- Soak Bengal gram and green gram overnight.
- Cook in a pressure cooker till tender.
- Add salt, red chilli powder, cumin powder, mango powder to the pulse and mix well.
- Apply the green chutney and khatti-meethi chutney to the inner sides of the bread slice.
- Stuff the filling between the bread slices.

Nutritive Value

Calories	-	247	kcal
Proteins	-	12.61	gm
Fats	-	1.85	gm
Iron	-	2.58	mg
Calcium	-	84.4	mg
Phosphorous	-	159.5	mg
Fibre	-	2.06	gm
Vitamin-C	-	0.75	mg
B-carotene	-	496	µg

6. LOW CALORIE FOODS [APPROX. 100 KCAL]

Vegetable Puda

Serving size: 2 number (50 gm)

Ingredients

Gram flour	- 20 gm
Onion	- 5 gm
Tomato	- 10 gm
Butter	- 2.5 gm
Salt	- to taste
Red chilli powder	- to taste
Cumin seed powder	- to taste

Preparation Steps

➤ Mix the gram flour, salt, red chilli powder and cumin powder with enough water to make a batter of dropping consistency.
➤ Add the finely chopped onion and tomatoes to the batter.
➤ Grease a griddle [tawa] with some butter and heat.
➤ Spread a little batter on the hot tawa.
➤ Cook until brown on the underside. Turn and cook on the other side.
➤ Serve hot with coriander chutney or tomato ketchup.

Nutritive Value

Calories	-	99.45	kcal
Proteins	-	3.6	gm
Fats	-	3.58	gm
Iron	-	1.04	mg
Calcium	-	47.2	mg
Phosphorous	-	67.4	mg
Fibre	-	0.89	gm
Vitamin-C	-	3	mg
B-carotene	-	85.65	µg

Sandwich

Serving size: 1

Ingredients

Bread	-	30 gm
Tomato	-	20 gm
Cucumber	-	20 gm
Onion	-	15 gm

Preparation Steps

➤ Cut tomatoes, cucumber and onion into thin slices.
➤ Apply chutney on the inner sides of the bread slices.
➤ Place the sliced vegetables in between the bread slices and serve.

Nutritive Value

Calories	-	88.95	kcal
Proteins	-	2.87	gm
Fats	-	0.28	gm
Iron	-	0.75	mg
Calcium	-	20.9	mg
Phosphorous	-	18	mg
Fibre	-	0.39	gm
Vitamin-C	-	7.1	mg
B-carotene	-	72.45	µg

BOTTLE GOURD PATTIES

Serving size: 1 serving = 4 nos. = 67 gm. (4 cm. Each)

Ingredients

Bottle gourd	- 100 gm
Gram flour	- 20 gm
Potatoes, boiled	- 10 gm
Ginger-garlic paste	- to taste
Green chillies, finely chopped	- 2-3
Salt	- to taste
Turmeric powder	- to taste
Red chilli powder	- to taste
Cumin seeds powder	- to taste

Preparation Steps

> Grate the bottle gourd.
> Mash the boiled potatoes, add the ginger-garlic paste, finely chopped green chillies, turmeric powder, salt, red chilli powder and cumin seed powder and mix well.
> Add grated bottle gourd and gram flour to this mixture.
> Shape into small thick cakes.
> Place the cakes in a baking dish and bake in hot oven at 180°C for 15 to 20 minutes.
> Serve hot with tomato ketchup.

Nutritive Value

Calories	-	95.15	kcal
Proteins	-	3.92	gm
Fats	-	1.2	gm
Iron	-	2.93	mg
Calcium	-	61.62	mg
Phosphorous	-	80.4	mg
Fibre	-	1.76	gm
Vitamin-C	-	17.45	mg
B-carotene	-	36.95	µg

BAKED SAGO WADA

Serving size: 1 serving = 2 nos. (4 cm each)

Ingredients

Sago (sabudana)	- 15 gm
Potato	- 30 gm
Oil	- 2.5 ml
Green chillies, finely chopped	- 2-3 in number
Lemon juice	- to taste
Salt	- to taste

Preparation Steps

> Soak sago for 1-2 hours in warm water. After 2 hours drain out water and keep it overnight.
> Boil potatoes and mash them. Add salt, chopped green chillies and lemon juice to the mashed potatoes. Mix well and add sago to it.

- Make small balls out of this mixture.
- Place the balls in a greased baking dish and bake in a hot oven at 200°C for 15-20 minutes.
- Serve hot with tomato ketchup or *khatti-meethi* chutney.

Nutritive Value

Calories	-	104.25	kcal
Proteins	-	0.51	gm
Fats	-	2.56	gm
Iron	-	0.339	mg
Calcium	-	4.5	mg
Phosphorous	-	13.5	mg
Fibre	-	0.12	gm
Vitamin-C	-	5.1	mg
B-carotene	-	7.2	µg
Niacin	-	0.36	mg

BHEL

Serving size: 1 serving = 1 cup = 72 gm.

Ingredients

Puffed rice	-	25 gm
Onion	-	15 gm
Tomato	-	20 gm
Potato	-	05 gm
Coriander	-	05 gm
Red chilli powder	-	to taste
Turmeric powder	-	to taste
Salt	-	to taste
Mustard seeds	-	to taste
Chat masala	-	to taste

Preparation Steps

- Heat and fry mustard seeds until they begin to crackle oil.
- Add red chilli powder, turmeric powder to the oil and then immediately add puffed rice to it.
- Add salt and mix well. Continue heating until they become crispy and crunchy.
- Finely chop the onion, tomato, boiled potato and coriander.
- Add the puffed rice to this and mix well.
- Add salt, chat masala and serve.

Nutritive Value

Calories	-	230	kcal
Proteins	-	6.6	gm
Fats	-	1.75	gm
Iron	-	7.31	mg
Calcium	-	217.95	mg
Phosphorous	-	168.82	mg
Fibre	-	5.07	gm
Vitamin-C	-	97.12	mg
B-carotene	-	385.92	µg

STEPS FOR KHATTI-MEETHI CHUTNEY

Ingredients

Dates	- 10 gm
Tamarind	- 20 gm
Red chilli powder	- 1/4 tsp
Coriander powder	- 1/4 tsp
Salt	- ½ tsp

Preparation Steps

- Seed the dates and tamarind.
- Soak in warm water for 1-2 hours.

> Blend the contents in a liquidiser and boil for a few minutes after adding red chilli powder, salt and coriander powder.

Steps for Green Chutney

Ingredients

Coriander leaves	- 50 gm
Green chillies	- 10 gm
Garlic	- 5 gm
Salt	- 1 tsp
Cumin seeds powder	- 2.5 gm
Lemon juice	- 10 ml
Water	- 10 ml

Preparation Steps

> Wash all the ingredients in running water.
> Cut the green chillies, garlic into small pieces and finely chop the coriander.
> Blend the contents in the liquidiser with all the ingredients mention above.

7. HIGH CALCIUM FOOD

Palak Sarsoon Puda

Serving size: 3 medium sizes

Ingredients

Palak	- 15 gm
Sarsoon	- 15 gm
Wheat flour	- 40 gm
Curd	- 50 gm
Oil	- 10 gm
Garlic, grated	- 1-2 flakes
Red chilli powder	- 1 tsp
Turmeric powder	- ½ tsp
Cumin	- ½ tsp
Salt	- to taste

Preparation Steps

> Remove stalks from palak and sarsoon.
> Chop and wash them.
> Add chopped palak, sarsoon, grated garlic, red chilli powder, turmeric powder, cumin, salt into wheat flour.
> Add water and make dough and divide the dough into three equal portions.
> Make round shaped parathas and shallow fry it.
> Serve hot with tomato chutney or green chutney.

Nutritive Value

Calories	- 273	kcal
Proteins	- 8.06	gm
Fats	- 13.69	gm
Iron	- 4.73	mg
Calcium	- 130	mg
Phosphorous	- 211	mg
Fibre	- 1.0	gm
Vitamin-C	- 21.54	mg
B-carotene	- 893	µg

Rabdi

Serving Size: 1 serving

Ingredients

Skimmed milk	- 350 ml
Sugar	- 20 gm
Almonds	- 05 gm
Pistachionuts	- 05 gm

Preparation Steps

- Pour milk in a pan.
- Let it boil until it thickens in consistency.
- Now add sugar and nuts.
- Serve chilled.

Nutritive Value

Calories	- 245.15 kcal
Proteins	- 10.8 gm
Fats	- 5.92 gm
Iron	- 1.36 mg
Calcium	- 440.90 mg
Phosphorous	- 341.60 mg
Fibre	- 0.19 gm
Vitamin-C	- 3.5 mg
B-carotene	- 7.20 µg

Gajar Ka Halwa

Serving size: 1 serving

Ingredients

Carrots	- 100 gm
Milk	- 150 ml
Sugar	- 10 gm

Preparation Steps

- Wash carrots and grate them.
- Pour milk into a pan.
- Add the grated carrots in the milk.
- Add sugar to the mixture.
- Cook this on a low flame until the milk is absorbed.
- Serve hot.

Nutritive Value

Calories	- 204.8 kcal
Proteins	- 7.35 gm
Fats	- 9.95 gm
Iron	- 1.56 mg
Calcium	- 396.2 mg
Phosphorous	- 725.10 mg
Fibre	- 1.20 gm
Vitamin-C	- 4.5 mg
B-carotene	- 1962 µg

Til Laddo

Serving size: 2 small size laddoos

Ingredients

Til seeds	- 25 gm
Groundnut	- 05 gm
Jaggery	- 20 gm

Preparation Steps

- Clean and roast the til seeds.
- Roast groundnuts and remove the skin.
- Grind them into fine powder.
- Add jaggery and mix well.
- Shape them into rounds.

Nutritive Value

Calories	- 245.00 kcal
Proteins	- 5.91 gm
Fats	- 12.82 gm
Iron	- 2.96 mg
Calcium	- 383.00 mg
Phosphorous	- 168.00 mg
Fibre	- 0.87 gm
Vitamin-C	- 0 mg
B-carotene	- 16.85 µg

Appendices

Appendix 1
A. Standard Weight and Height Tables

Age (years)	Boys Height (cm)	Boys Weight (kg)	Girls Height (cm)	Girls Weight (kg)
1.0	76.1	10.2	74.3	9.5
1.5	82.4	11.5	80.9	10.8
2.0	85.6	12.3	84.5	11.8
2.5	90.4	13.5	89.5	13
3.0	99.1	15.7	93.9	14.1
3.5	99.1	15.7	97.9	15.1
4.0	102.9	16.7	101.6	16.0
4.5	106.6	17.7	105.1	16.8
5.0	109.9	18.7	108.4	17.7
5.5	113.1	19.7	111.6	18.6
6.0	116.1	20.7	114.6	19.5
6.5	119.0	21.7	117.6	20.6
7.0	121.7	22.9	120.6	21.8
7.5	124.4	24.0	123.5	23.3
8.0	127.0	25.3	126.4	24.8
8.5	129.6	26.7	129.3	26.6
9.0	132.2	28.1	132.2	28.5
9.5	134.8	29.7	135.2	30.5
10.0	137.5	31.4	138.3	32.5
10.5	140.3	33.3	141.5	34.7
11.0	143.3	35.3	144.8	37.0
11.5	146.4	37.5	148.2	39.2
12.0	149.7	39.8	151.5	41.5
12.5	153.0	42.3	154.6	43.8
13.0	156.5	45	157.1	46.1
13.5	159.9	47.8	159.0	48.3
14.0	163.1	50.8	160.0	50.3
14.5	166.2	53.8	161.2	52.1
15.0	169.0	56.7	161.8	53.7
15.5	171.5	59.5	162.1	55.0
16.0	173.5	62.1	162.4	55.9
16.5	175.2	64.4	162.7	56.4
17.0	176.2	66.3	163.1	56.7
17.5	176.7	67.8	163.4	56.7
18.0	176.8	68.9	163.7	56.6

Ref: National Centre for Health Statistics (NCHS), USA, Standards.

B. Mean Height-Weight Tables for Well-To-Do Children and Adults

Age (years)	Male Height (cm)	Male Weight (kg)	Female Height (cm)	Female Weight (kg)
At Birth	50.5	3.3	49.9	3.2
3 months	61.1	6.0	60.2	5.4
6 months	67.8	7.8	66.6	7.2
9 months	72.3	9.2	71.1	8.6
1+	80.07	10.54	78.09	9.98
2+	90.01	12.51	87.93	11.67
3+	98.36	14.78	96.21	13.79
4+	104.70	16.12	104.19	15.85
5+	113.51	19.33	112.24	18.67
6+	118.90	22.14	117.73	21.56
7+	123.32	24.46	122.65	24.45
8+	127.86	26.42	127.22	25.97
9+	133.63	30.00	133.08	29.82
10+	138.45	32.29	138.90	33.58
11+	143.35	35.26	145.00	37.17
12+	148.91	38.78	150.98	42.97
13+	154.94	42.88	153.44	44.54
14+	161.70	48.26	155.04	46.70
15+	165.33	52.15	155.98	48.75
16+	168.40	55.54	156.00	49.75
17+	173.00	57.91	-	-
18+	172.05	58.38	-	-
19+	172.14	58.90	-	-
20+	171.75	59.64	-	-
21+	172.40	59.74	-	-
22+	171.63	60.14	-	-

Ref: Indian Council of Medical Research (ICMR), 2002.

C (i). Standard Weight (kg) for Men at Various Heights and Ages

Height cm	Age (years)						
	20	25	30	35	40	45	50
148	42.7	44.2	46.2	47.6	48.8	50.0	50.9
150	43.6	44.9	46.9	48.5	49.7	50.8	51.5
153	45.4	47.0	49.0	50.4	51.7	52.3	53.5
155	46.3	48.1	49.9	51.5	52.7	53.5	54.2
158	48.6	50.0	52.0	53.5	54.5	55.7	56.3
160	49.7	51.1	53.1	54.7	55.6	56.7	57.4
163	51.1	52.7	54.9	56.3	57.6	58.5	59.4
165	53.1	54.7	56.9	58.5	59.7	60.6	62.0
168	54.0	56.3	58.1	60.1	61.5	62.4	63.7
170	56.5	57.9	60.3	62.2	63.7	64.7	65.8
173	58.1	60.1	62.2	64.0	65.8	67.0	68.3
175	60.1	62.2	64.2	66.0	68.1	69.7	71.0
178	61.9	64.0	66.3	68.5	70.6	71.9	72.4
180	64.0	66.2	68.5	71.0	73.3	74.4	75.1
183	66.0	68.5	71.0	73.3	75.6	77.1	77.8

(ii) Standard Weight (kg) for Women at Various Heights and Ages

Height cm	Age (years)						
	20	25	30	35	40	45	50
148	38.6	41.0	42.6	44.0	45.1	46.3	47.1
150	40.3	41.6	43.5	44.8	46.0	47.0	47.7
153	41.9	43.5	45.3	46.6	47.9	48.4	49.5
155	42.8	44.3	46.2	47.7	48.8	49.5	50.1
158	44.9	46.3	48.1	49.5	50.4	51.6	52.1
160	46.0	47.3	49.9	50.6	51.5	52.4	53.0
163	47.3	48.8	50.8	52.1	52.2	54.1	54.9
165	49.1	50.6	52.6	54.1	55.3	56.0	57.3
168	50.0	52.1	53.8	55.6	56.8	57.7	59.0

Ref: F. P. Antia & Philip Abraham, *Clinical Dietitics and Nutrition*, 1997, Oxford University Press, pp 496-97.

D. Recommended Dietary Allowances

Group	Particulars	Body weight	Net energy	Protein	Visible fat	Calcium	Iron	Vit A (ug/d)		Thia-mine	Ribo-flavin	Niacin	Pyri-doxin	Vit C	Free Folic Acid	Vit-B12
								Retinol	B Carotene							
		Kg	Kcal/d	g/d	g/d	mg/d	mg/d			mg/d	mg/d	mg/d	mg/d	mg/d	ug/d	ug/d
Man	Sedentary	60	2425	60	20	400	28	600	2400	1.2	1.4	16	2.0	40	100	1.0
	Moderate		2875							1.4	1.6	18				
	Heavy		3800							1.6	1.9	21				
Woman	Sedentary	50	1875	50	20	400	30	600	2400	0.9	1.1	12	2.0	40	100	1.0
	Moderate		2225							1.1	1.3	14				
	Heavy		2925							1.2	1.5	16				
	Pregnant	50	+300	+15	30	1000	38	600	2400	+0.2	+0.2	+2	2.5	40	400	1.0
	Lactating 0-6 m	50	+550	+25	45	1000	30	950	3800	+0.3	+0.3	+4	2.5	80	150	1.5
	6-12 m		+400	+18						+0.2	+0.2	+3				
Infants	0-6 m	5.4	108/Kg	2.05/Kg		500	-	350	1200	55ug/Kg	65ug/Kg	710ug/Kg	0.1	25	25	0.2
	6-12 m	8.6	98/Kg	1.65/Kg						50ug/Kg	60ug/Kg	650ug/Kg	0.4			
Children	1-3 years	12.2	1240	22	25	400	12	400	1600	0.6	0.7	8	0.9	40	30	0.2-1.0
	4-6 years	19.0	1690	30			18	400	2400	0.9	1.0	11			40	
	7-9 years	26.9	1950	41			26	600		1.0	1.2	13	1.6		60	
Boys	10-12 years	35.4	2190	54	22	600	34	600	2400	1.1	1.3	15	1.6	40	70	0.2-1.0
Girls	10-12 years	35.5	1970	57			19			1.0	1.2	13				
Boys	13-15 years	47.8	2450	70	22	600	41	600	2400	1.2	1.5	16	2.0	40	100	0.2-1.0
Girls	13-15 years	46.7	2060	65			28			1.0	1.2	14				
Boys	16-18 years	57.1	2640	78	22	500	50	600	2400	1.3	1.6	17	2.0	40	100	0.2-1.0
Girls	16-18 years	49.9	2060	63			30			1.0	1.2	14				

Source: Nutritive Value of Indian Foods (NIN), ICMR, 2004.

E. Food Pyramid for Good Health

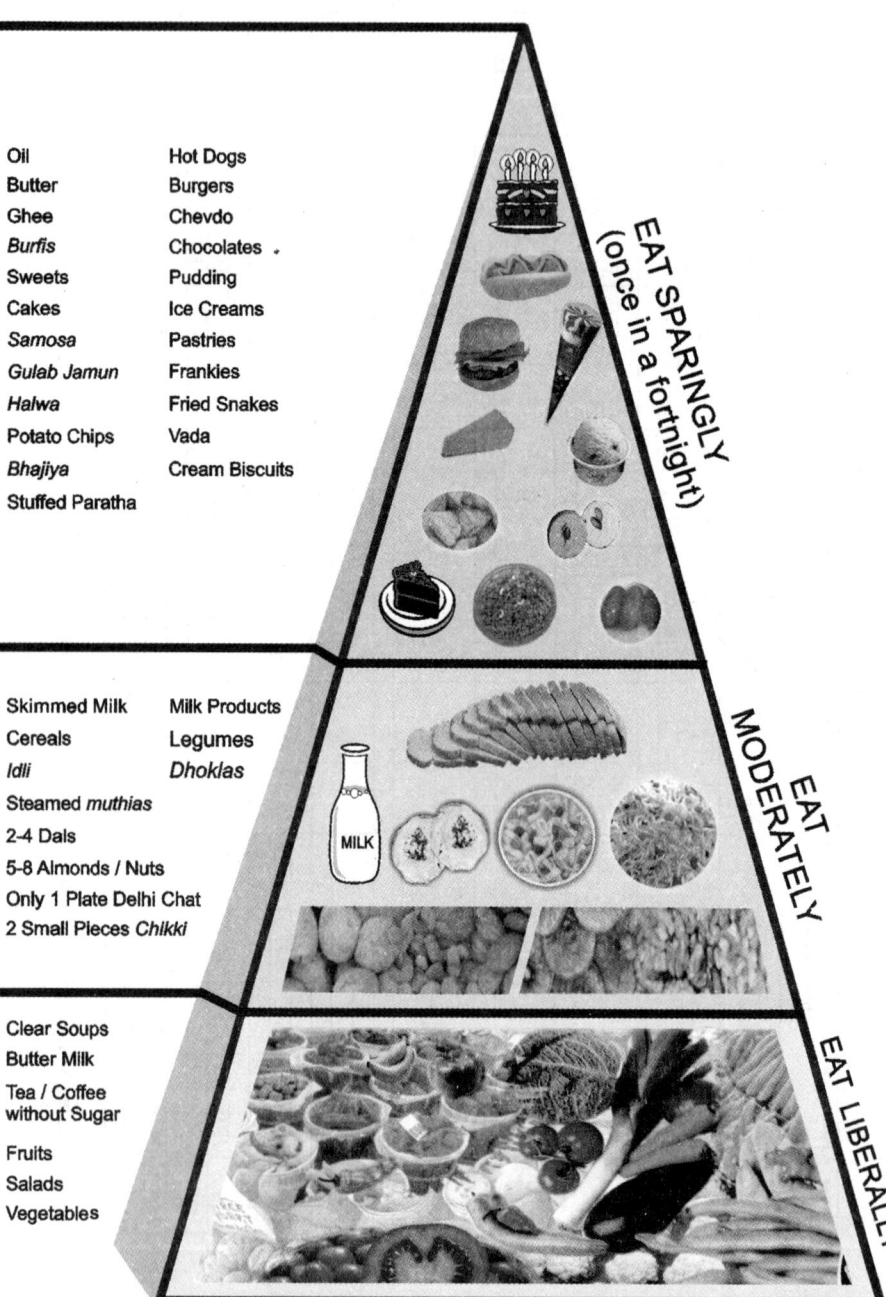

EAT SPARINGLY (once in a fortnight)
- Oil
- Butter
- Ghee
- *Burfis*
- Sweets
- Cakes
- *Samosa*
- *Gulab Jamun*
- *Halwa*
- Potato Chips
- *Bhajiya*
- Stuffed Paratha
- Hot Dogs
- Burgers
- Chevdo
- Chocolates
- Pudding
- Ice Creams
- Pastries
- Frankies
- Fried Snakes
- Vada
- Cream Biscuits

EAT MODERATELY
- Skimmed Milk
- Cereals
- *Idli*
- Steamed *muthias*
- 2-4 Dals
- 5-8 Almonds / Nuts
- Only 1 Plate Delhi Chat
- 2 Small Pieces *Chikki*
- Milk Products
- Legumes
- *Dhoklas*

EAT LIBERALLY
- Clear Soups
- Butter Milk
- Tea / Coffee without Sugar
- Fruits
- Salads
- Vegetables

F. Food Items Containing Energy
kcal / 100 gm of edible portion

Very High > 500	High 200 – 500	Moderate High 50 – 200	Low < 50
Ghee (900)	Sugar	Milk (buffalo – 117) (cow – 67)	Buttermilk (15)
Butter (720)	Honey	Curd	Skimmed milk liquid (29)
Hydrogenated oil (fortified) (900)	Jaggery	Meat & poultry Mutton (194) Pork (114)	Tomato (20)
Cooking oil (900)	Whole milk powder (496) Skimmed milk (357)	Fishes & sea foods	Pineapple (46)
Dry fruits (500 – 687)	Milk (*Khoa*) (421)	Fruits	Papaya (32)
	Beef meat	Potato (97)	Orange (48) Sweet lime (43)
	Raisins (308)	Peas, green	Figs, fresh (37)
	Apricot	Red gram, tender	Coconut water
	Black current	Fruits Banana (116) Apple (59) Dates (144) Mango (74) Pomegranate (65) Custard Apple (104)	Roots and tubers Radish (17) Beetroot (43) Carrots (48)
	Dry dates	Chicken (98)	
	Coconut, fresh	Egg (173)	
	Coconut milk	Fowl (109)	
	Cereals		
	Pulses		

G. Food Items Containing Proteins
gm / 100 gm of edible portion

Very High > 20 gms	High 15 – 20 gms	Moderate High 10 gms	Low <5 gm
Bengal gram	Bengal gram (Whole)	Red gram (Tender)	Butter milk
Black gram	*Chenna*	Rice	Milk
Cow pea	Wheat Flour	Rice flakes	Banana
Green gram	Semolina	Rice puffed	Apple
Red beans	Coriander	Cauliflower, green	Cherries
Red gram	Egg (Hen)	Bengal gram leaves	Brinjal
Soyabean	Gingelly seeds	Carrot leaves	*Amla*
Cheese	Walnut	Curry leaves	Cucumber
Khoa		Colocasia	Sapota
Skimmed milk powder		Tamarind leaves	Lady's finger
Almond			Maize (tender)
Cashewnut			Cabbage
Groundnut			Sugarcane juice
Mustard seeds			Spinach
Niger seeds			Mint
Watermelon seeds			Coconut milk

H. Food Items Containing Crude Fibres
gm / 100 gm of edible portion

Very High 9 - 15 gms	High 3 – 7 gms	Low 1 – 3 gms	Very Low Nil gms
Sanwa millet	Coriander leaves	Maize (dry)	Fishes & sea foods
Gingelly seeds (2.9)	Red beans (4.8) Soyabean (3.7)	*Bajra* (1.2)	
Niger seeds (10.9)	Red gram tender (6.2)	*Jowar* (1.6)	
Coconut dry (6.6)	Guava (5.2)	Wheat (1.2)	Meat & poultry
	Pomegranate	Fenugreek leaves (1.1)	
	Drumstick	Almond (1.7) Cashewnut (1.3)	Milk & milk products
	Coconut (fresh)	Bengal gram (3.9)	
	Amla	Red gram dal (1.5)	Fats & edible oils
	Woodapple	Black gram (1.9)	
		Leafy veg.	Sugar
		Fruits	
			Rice flakes (0.7) Puffed rice (0.3) Semolina (0.2)

I. Food Items Containing Fat
gm / 100 gm of edible portion

Very High 50 – 100	High 40 – 50	Moderate High 20 – 30	Low < 5
Almond (58.9)	Coconut (fresh) (41.6)	*Khoa* (buffalo milk) (31.2)	Cereals
Coconut dry (62.3)	Coconut (milk)	*Khoa* (buffalo milk, skimmed) (1.6)	Pulses
Sunflower seed	Gingelly seeds (43.3)	Cheese (25.1)	Leafy veg.
Walnut (64.5) Cashewnut (46.9)	Groundnut (40.1)	Soyabean (19.5)	Roots & tubers
Watermelon seed	Niger seeds (*kala til*) (39)		Other veg.
Pistachionut (53.5)			
Butter (72.9)			
Ghee (100)			
All brands of oil (100)			

J. Potassium (K) Rich Foods
mg per 100 gms of edible portion

Very-High > 1000	High 1000 – 500	Moderate 500 – 100	Low < 100
Cow pea (1131)	Pulses	Cereals	Wheat, semolina (83)
Green gram dal (1150)	Tapioca chips, dried (764)	Red gram, tender (463)	Peas, green (79)
Moth beans (1096)	Colocasia (550)	Leafy vegetables	Fenugreek leaves (31)
Red gram, whole red gram, dal (1104)		Roots & tubers	Lettuce (33)
		Other vegetables	Radish, pink (10)
		Condiments & spices	Beetroot (43)
		Fruits	Arrowroot flour (20)
		Meat & poultry	Bottle gourd (87)
		Milk & other products	Broad beans (39)
			Cucumber (50)
			Field beans (47)
			Mango, green (83)
			Parwar (83)
			Ridge gourd
			Snake gourd
			Tinda, tender (24)
			Nuts & oilseeds (0)
			Apple (75)
			Banana ripe (88)
			Guava country (91)
			Jambu fruit (55)
			Orange (9.3)
			Papaya ripe (69)
			Pears (96)
			Pineapple (37)
			Rose apple (50)
			Milk, buffalo's (90)

K. Sodium (Na) Rich Foods
mg per 100 gm edible portion

High > 30	Moderate 30 – 10	Low < 10
Pulses & legumes	Cereals	Yam
Maize, tender (51.7)	Roots & tubers	Sweet potato
Leafy vegetables	Snake gourd	Tapioca chips, dried
Arrowroot	Cherries, red	Other vegetables
Beetroot	Apple (28)	Condiments & spices
Carrot	Jambu, fruit (26.2)	Fruits
Radish, pink	Mango, ripe (26)	*Amla* (5)
Radish, white	Watermelon (27.3)	Cape gooseberry (0.9)
Broad beans	Milk, buffalo's	Guava, country (5.5)
Cauliflower	Milk, goat's	
Field beans, tender		
Jack, tender		
Pink beans		
Tinda, tender		
Tomato, green		
Pineapple (34.7)		
Banana, ripe (36.6)		
Lichi (124.9)		
Musk melon (104.6)		
Meat & poultry		
Milk, cow's (73)		
Curd, cow's milk (32)		
Rose apple		

L. Iron Rich Food
per 100 gm of edible portion

High > 10 mg	Moderate 2 – 10 mg	Low < 2 mg
Rice flakes (20)	*Bajra* (8)	All other cereals & grains
Amaranth tristis (38.5)	*Jowar* (4.2)	Cabbage (0.8)
Bengal gram leaves (23.8)	Rice, puffed (6.6)	
Cauliflower green (40.5)	Sanwa millet (5)	Spinach (1.5)
Mustard leaves (16.3)	Wheat, whole (5.3)	All other roots & tubers
Rape leaves (12.3)	Wheat flour refined (2.7)	Most vegetables
Raddish leaves (18)	Bengal gram dal (5.3)	Most fruits
Niger seeds (56.7)	Bengal gram, roasted (9.5)	All fish & other sea food
Garden Cress seeds (100)	All other pulses	Most meat & poultry
	All other leafy vegetables	Fat & Oil
	Kankoda (4.6)	Sugar
	Coconut dry (7.8)	Milk
	Mackerel (4.5) Mutton muscle (2.5)	Condiment & spices

M. Calcium Content Food
mgs / 100 gm of edible portion

Very High > 200	High 100 – 200	Moderate High 50 – 100	Low < 50
Fenugreek leaves (395)	Bengal gram	Green gram, whole	All cereals
Almond (230)	Shepu	Moth beans	
Gingelly seeds (1450)	Dates, dried	Red beans	Roots and tubers
Coconut dry	*Phalsa*	Soya bean	
Milk (buffalo's) (210)	Wood apple	Black gram dal	Sugar
Skimmed milk powder (1370)	Milk (cow's)	Coriander leaves	Bengal gram (roasted)
Drumstick leaves (440)	Curd	Spinach	Bengal gram dal
Colocasia leaves (460)		Walnut	Cow pea
Radish leaves (265)	Pistachionut	Cashewnut	Green gram dal
Crab (1606)			Green gram, whole
Cheese (790)			Field, bean dry
Khoa (650)			Lentil
Khoa, skimmed milk, buffalo (990)			Peas (green)
			Peas (dry)
			Peas (roasted)
			Red gram, dal
			Red gram, tender
			Groundnut
			Other vegetables
			Fruits except wood apple, dates (dried)

N. Comprehensive Food Exchange List

Sr. No	Exchange	Amount g Raw food	Measure Raw food	Protein g	CHO g	Fat g	Kcal	Na mg	K mg
1	Milk	250	1C	8	12	10	170	40	350
2-A	Veg - A	100	½ C	Neg.	Neg.	Neg.	Neg.	30	100
2-B	Veg - B	100-150	½ C	2	7	Neg.	40	50	200
3	Fruit	80-100	1 port.	Neg.	10	Neg.	40	12	80
4	Cereal	20	3 tbsp	2	15	Neg.	70	3	40
5-A	Meat	40	2pc or 1 egg	7	Neg.	5	70	50	80
5-B	Pulse	30	3 tbc	7	17	Neg.	100	10	200
7	Fat	5	1 t	0	0	5	45	Neg.	Neg.

O. Milk Exchange
8 gm. Protein, 12 gm. Carbohydrate, 10 gm. Fat, 170 kcal.

Foodstuffs	Amount g	Protein g	CHO g	Fat g	Kcal	Na mg	K mg
Milk, cow	250	8	11.5	10.3	168	40	350
Milk, buffalo	185	8	9.3	16.3	216	35	166
Skim milk, liquid	250	8	14.7	Neg.	93	51	448
Whole milk powder	31	8	11.8	8	154	83 (Amul)	222
Curds	258	8	7.7	10.3	155	83(118)	335 315
Skim milk powder	21	8	10.7	Neg.	75	112(108)	195 (Vita) 366
Chenna, cow	44	8	0.5	9.2	117	(82)19 DMS toned	(332) 32 DMS toned
Cheese	33	8	2.1	8.4	115	429 (364)	15 (Amul)
Khoa, buffalo	55	8	11.3	17.2	231	-	-
Khoa, cow	40	8	10.0	10.4	165	-	-
Khoa, skim, buffalo	34	8	9.1	0.6	72	-	-

DMS/Mother dairy milk has 100 mg. Na and 290 mg. K per 250 g. Butter milk values same as for curds.

Add two fat exchanges because these forms of milk contain no fat.

P. Vegetable Exchange
Negligible carbohydrate, negligible protein and negligible fat
2 exchanges of veg A calculated as 1 exchange of veg B

Foodstuff	Carbohydrate %	Na mg	K mg
Bathua leaves	2.9	–	
Bottle gourd	2.5	20	57
Cucumber	2.5	10	50
Ghosalas	2.9	–	
Lettuce	2.5	59	33
Mustard leaves	3.2	18	220
Parwar	2.2	3	83
Radish leaves	2.4	–	–
Radish, white	3.4	33	138
Ridge gourd	3.4	3	50
Snake gourd	3.3	25	34
Spinach	2.9	59	206
Tinda	3.4	35	24

Q. Vegetable B Exchange
7 gm. carbohydrate, 2 gm. protein, negligible fat, 40 kcal

Foodstuff	Weight g	CHO g	Protein g	Kcal	Na mg	K mg
Amaranth	115	7	4.6	52	264	392
Beetroot	80	7	1.4	34	48	34
Bitter gourd	167	7	2.7	42	3	253
Brinjal	175	7	2.7	42	5	350
Broad beans	97	7	4.4	47	42	37
Cabbage	152	7	2.7	41	21	173
Capsicum	163	7	2.1	39	–	–
Carrot	66	7	0.6	32	24	71
Cauliflower	175	7	4.5	53	92	241
Colocasia leaves	103	7	4.3	58	–	–
Drumstick	192	7	4.8	50	–	–
Coriander leaves	111	7	3.7	40	65	284
Fenugreek leaves	117	7	3.1	57	90	36
French beans	156	7	2.6	41	6	187
Jackfruit, tender	75	7	1.9	38	26	246
Kholkhol	184	7	22.1	39	206	68
Lady's finger	100	7	2.0	38	8	112
Mint leaves	121	7	5.0	58	–	–
Onion, small	56	7	1.0	33	2	71
Peas	44	7	3.2	41	3	35
Pumpkin	152	7	2.1	38	9	211
Tomato	194	7	1.7	30	25	283
Turnip	113	7	0.6	33	66 (H)	269 (H)

R. Fruit Exchange
10 g. carbohydrate, negligible protein and fat, 40 kcal

Foodstuff	Weight g	CHO g
Amla	74	10
Apricot	86	10
Apple	75	10
Banana	37	10
Cherries	72	10
Dates, fresh	30	10
Grape Fruit	143	10
Grapes	61	10
Guava	80	10
Lemon, big (*nimbu*)	92	10
Lichi	73	10
Lime, sweet (*malta*)	128	10
Lime, sweet (*mausambi*)	107	10
Loquat	104	10
Mango, ripe	59	10
Musk melon	286	10
Orange	92	10
Papaya	139	10
Pear	84	10
Pineapple	93	10
Plums	90	10
Pomegranate	69	10
Raspberry	86	10
Raisins	13	10
Sapota	47	10
Water melon	303	10

S. Cereal Exchange
15 gm. carbohydrate, 2 gm. protein, negligible fat, 70 kcal

Foodstuff	Weight g	CHO g	Protein g	Kcal	Na mg	K mg
Bajra	22	15	2.6	79	2	68
Barley	22	15	2.5	72	4	56
Bread, white	29	15	2.3	69	152	32
Bread, brown	31	15	2.7	76	158	81
Biscuits, salty	28	15	1.8	150	185	18
Biscuits, sweet	21	15	1.3	96	43 (H)	27 (H)
Cake, cream						
Cake, sponge		15	7.9	226	54	83
Jowar	21	15	2.1	73	1	26
Cornflakes	18	15	1.4	72	181	22
Maize, dry	23	15	2.5	70	4	22
Oatmeal	24	15	3.3	90	Neg	85
Ragi	21	15	1.5	69	2	86
Rice	19	15	1.3	66	2	13
Rice, flakes	20	15	1.3	65	2	31
Rice, puffed	20	15	2.1	66	-	-
Semolina	20	15	2.1	70	4	16

T. Meat and Pulse Exchange
A Meat Exchange
7 g protein, 5 g fat, negligible carbohydrate, 70 kcals

Foodstuff	Weight g	Protein g	Fat g	Kcal	Na mg	K mg
Egg yolk	39	7	11.3	138	20	38
Egg	53	7	7.0	81	65	63
Egg white	58	7	-	26	85	81
Fowl	27	7	0.2	29	12 (H)	110 (H)
Goat meat	32	7	1.2	38	-	-
Goat liver	35	7	1.1	38	26	58
Sheep liver	35	7	2.6	53	-	-
Mutton, muscle	3837	7	5.1	73	13	103
Pork	37	7	1.7	43	17 (H)	148 (H)
Crab	63	7	6.1	106	231	171
Hilsa	32	7	6.2	87	17	58
Katla	35	7	0.8	39	17	53
Pomfret	41	7	0.5	33	-	-
Pawn	37	7	0.4	32	24	96

Table contd...

Foodstuff	Weight g	Protein g	Fat g	Kcal	Na mg	K mg
Sardines	32	7	0.6	34	251(H)	139 (H) (canned in oil)
Rohu	42	7	0.6	41	42	121
Singhara	34	7	1.0	53	-	-
Chenna	38	7	7.9	101	16.87 (DMS toned)	28 (DMS toned)
Cheese	29	7	7.3	101	377 340	32 (Amul) 13
Chenna, buffalo	52	7	1.2	162	-	-
Protinex	12.5	7	-	28	-	-
Sausages	80	7	23.0	273	616 (H)	126 (H)

B Pulse Exchange

Foodstuff	Weight g	Protein g	Fat g	CHO g	Kcal	Na mg	K mg
Bengal gram, whole	41	7	2.2	25	148	13	331
Bengal gram, dal	34	7	1.8	20	125	25	245
Black gram, dal	29	7	0.4	17	101	11	232
Cow pea	29	7	0.3	16	94	7	328
Green gram, whole	29	7	0.4	16	97	7	236
Green gram, dal	28	7	0.3	17	101	8	332
Lentil	29	7	0.2	16	96	12	182
Bean, dry	35	7	0.4	20	105	7	254
Red beans	30	7	0.5	18	105	3	295 (Red dry)
Red gram, dal	31	7	0.5	18	104	10	342
Soyabean	16	7	3.2	3.4	70	(4)	270
Nutri nuggets	14	7	0.1	4.2	48	Neg.	254

Sprouted group gram provides 0.63 B1, 0.6 B2, 4.1 mg. Niacin and 82 mg of vitamin C when 100 g dal is soaked and sprouted.

U. Fat Exchange

Provides negligible carbohydrate and protein and fat 5 g, kcal 45

Foodstuff	Weight g	Protein g	Fat g	Kcal	Na mg	K mg
Egg yolk	39	7	11.3	138	20	38
Butter (salted)	6	0	5	45	59	(2)
Ghee	5	0	5	45	-	-
Hydrogenated oil	5	0	5	45	-	-
Almonds	8	1.7	5	53	tr	62
Cooking oil	5	0	5	45	-	-
Cashewnuts	11	2.0	5	66	(2)	(51)
Coconut, dry	8	0.3	5	53	-	-
Coconut, fresh	12	0.5	5	53	2	52
Gingelly seeds	12	2.2	5	58	-	-
Groundnut, roasted	13	3.4	5	74	tr	92
Walnuts	8	1.3	5	55	tr	36
Bacon	10	3.5	5	60	102	24
Cream, light 20%	25	Neg.	5	45	11	21
Cream, 40%	15	Neg.	5	45	-	-
Mayonnaise	6	Neg.	5	45	-	-

V. Miscellaneous - Per 100 gm. edible portion

Foodstuff	Na mg	K mg
Baking powder	8220	170
Bread crumbs	740	150
Chocolate (bitter)	4	830
Cocoa powder	6	1522
Soy sauce	7320	370
Beer	7	25
Arrowroot flour	3	20
Cornstarch	-	4
Tapioca	3	18
Honey	5	31
Yeast (baker's)	10	610
Gin	1	2
Table wine	5	92
Coffee powder	72	3256
Marmalade	14	33
Mayonnaise	597	54
Garlic	19	529
Salt (table)	38800	tr
Jam	12	88

Appendix 2
Standard Measurements

Product	Volume/ Household measures	Grams
Pulses	1 cup	200
Gram flour (sifted)	1 cup	90
Green grams	1 cup	200
Channa	1 cup	200
Rajma	1 cup	200
Flour (sifted)	1 cup	100
Milk (liquid)	1 cup	200
Milk powder	1 cup	138
Milk powder	1 tablespoon	8.4
Condensed milk	1 cup	220
Khoa	1 cup	200
Paneer	1 cup	150
Cream	1 cup	200
Curd	1 cup	200
Butter	1 cup	227
Butter	1 tablespoon	14
Cocoa powder	1 tablespoon	7.2
Baking powder	1 tablespoon	3
Sugar (granulated)	1 cup	200
Sugar (granulated)	1 tablespoon	15
Water	1 cup	200
Jaggery	1 cup	200
Yeast, dry	1 tablespoon	4
Salt	1 teaspoon	5
Soda	1 teaspoon	3
Cornflour	1 teaspoon	10
Rice	1 cup	200
Oil	1 cup	180
Oil	1 tablespoon	12
Ghee (melted)	1 cup	180
Ghee (melted)	1 tablespoon	12
Groundnuts	1 cup	200
Nuts (chopped)	1 cup	200

1 cup = 200 ml ½ teaspoon = 2.5 ml ½ cup = 100 ml
¼ teaspoon = 1.25 ml ¼ cup = 50 ml 1 tablespoon = 15 ml
1 teaspoon = 5 ml

Appendix 3

Common Terminologies and Phrases Associated with Obesity

In order to understand obesity, a few other terms need to be discussed which are as follows:

Desirable Body Weight: The desirable weight of a person is empirically decided by using the height, weight, age and sex for the respective individual. Height-weight tables for normal individuals are provided in the Appendix (I). Using these tables the desirable weight can be calculated.

Referring to these tables one need not necessarily adhere to the exact weight but a ± of 2 kg should fall within the acceptable range.

The advantages of maintaining desirable body weight include improved immune system as well as it prevents occurrence of chronic degenerative diseases.

Overweight: Overweight is the condition of the body whereby there is a limited increase in the weight of the body. This increase is limited up to 20% of the desirable weight.

Let the desirable weight of a person be 50 kg in relation to his age, height and sex. If this weight increases up to 60 kg (i.e. 50 × 1.2 = 60), then he can be considered as overweight.

Underweight: Underweight is the condition of the body whereby there is remarkable decrease in the weight of the body. This decrease is 10% or more than the desirable weight.

Let the desirable weight of a person be 50 kg in relation to his age, height and sex. If the weight decreases below 45 kg. (i.e. 50 X 0.9 = 45), he is considered underweight.

Obesity: Obesity is a condition of the body where there is a remarkable increase in the weight of the body and this increase is more than 20% of the desirable weight.

Let the desirable weight of the person be 50 kg in relation to his age, height and sex. If the weight is more than 60 kg he will be considered as obese.

The terms overweight and obesity are not always understood in its true sense and are often considered as synonyms. However scientifically these two terms are different and should not be confused. Refer figure 1.

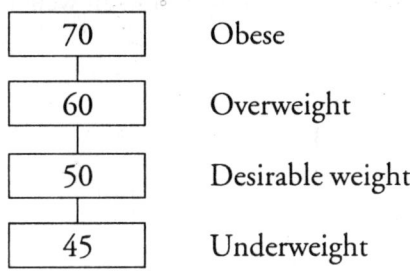

Figure 1

Obesity in itself is not a disease but a disorder in the body. It may be described as an agent, which leads to "Bundle of Diseases" resulting in a significant impairment of health. It invites various complications like diabetes mellitus, hypertension, cancer, heart disease, arthritis and sometimes leads to premature deaths.

Morbid Obesity: Morbid obesity can be defined as being 40-100% heavier than your ideal body weight. A BMI of greater than 39 indicates morbid obesity. Over 30 serious medical complications can arise as direct result of obesity.

Energy Balance: This can be explained by understanding the mechanism of kinetics of body weight. The energy-giving foods are called fuel foods, which are necessary for the growth and development of the body.

The energy consumed by the body from the foods is called *energy intake*, while the energy spend by the body to perform various functions is called *energy output*. When these two are nearly equal the body weight is maintained.

Positive Energy Balance: The condition in which the energy input exceeds the energy output leading to accumulation of excess fat in the body, which ultimately results in increased body weight.

Negative Energy Balance: The condition in which the energy output exceeds the energy input leading to burning of body fat, which ultimately results in weight loss.

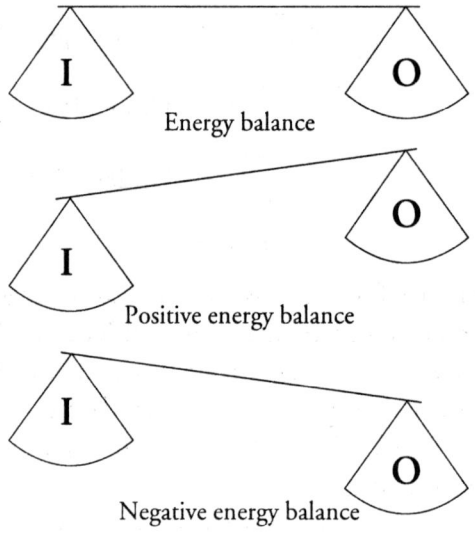

Where I = Energy Input
       O = Energy Output

Figure 2

Adaptive Thermogenesis: Changes in the amount of energy expended in response to changes in circumstance, such as over or underfeeding, changes in ambient temperature, or trauma are referred to as adaptive thermogenesis.

Anorexia Nervosa: An eating disorder characterised by extreme weight loss, poor body image, and irrational fears of weight gain and obesity.

or

An eating disorder characterised by self-starvation, a distorted body image, and low body weight.

Appetite: The desire to eat; a pleasant sensation that is aroused by the thoughts of the taste and enjoyment of food.

or

The non-physiological factors that signal the selection and consumption of specific foods.

Artificial Sweeteners: A chemically manufactured sweetner that differs from simple sugars in chemical structure and often provides little or no energy when ingested.

Balanced Diet: A balanced diet is one which provides all the nutrients in required amounts and proper proportions. It can be easily achieved through blend of four basic food groups.

A balanced diet should provide around 60-70% of total calories from carbohydrates, preferably starch, about 10-12% from proteins and 20-25% from fat.

Basal Metabolic Rate (BMR): A measure of the minimum amount of energy that an awake but resting body needs to maintain itself.

Behaviour Modification: A process used to gradually and permanently change habitual behaviour.

Binge Eating: The consumption of a large amount of food in a small amount of time.

Binge-eating Disorder: An eating disorder characterised by periodic binge eating, which normally is not followed by vomiting or the use of laxatives. People must experience eating binges twice a week on an average for over six months to qualify for the diagnosis.

Body Mass Index: An index of weight in relation to height that is used to compare body size with a standard, it is equal to body weight (in kgs) divided by height (in meters squared).

Brown Adipose Tissue: A type of fat tissue that has a greater number of mitochondria than the more common white adipose tissue. It can waste energy by producing heat and is believed to be responsible for some of the change in energy expenditure in adaptive thermogenesis.

Calorie: A unit of measure of the amount of energy supplied by food. Also known as kilocalories, or the large calorie with a capital 'C'.

or

The amount of heat required to raise the temperature of 1 gm of water by 1°C; equal to 4.18 joules.

Diet History: A diet history is a less clearly defined procedure that collects information about dietary habits and patterns. It may include a history of nutritional habits.

Food Labels: Food labels are another tool that can be used in diet planning. They are designed to help the consumers make food choices by providing information about the nutrient composition of foods and about how a food fits into the overall diet.

Gene: A gene is a segment of DNA that provides the blueprint for the synthesis of or codes for protein.

Hunger: An unpleasant physical and psychological sensation (weakness, stomach pains, irritability) that lead people to acquire and ingest food.

or

Internal signals that stimulate one to acquire and consume food.

Hypothalamus: The region of the brain that regulates food intake and energy expenditure.

Leptin: Leptin is a protein hormone produced by the fat cells and released into the circulation where it travels to the hypothalamus.

Liposuction: A cosmetic procedure that removes localised fat deposits by vacuuming out the fat tissue.

Protein Sparing Modified Food: A very low kcalorie diet of high protein content designed to maximise the loss of fat and minimise the loss of protein from the body.

Recommended Dietary Allowances: Daily levels of nutrient intake that meet the needs of practically all healthy persons while decreasing the risk of certain chronic diseases.

Satiety: A feeling of fullness or of having had enough to eat.

Set or Setting Point: A level at which body fat or body weight seems to resist change despite changes in energy intake or output.

Syndrome X: A cluster of abnormalities including obesity, hypertriglyceridaemia, reduced level of HDL cholesterol, hyperinsulinemia, glucose intolerance and hypertension coupled with increased atherogenic small dense LDL particles elevated apo B concentrations and raised plasminogen activator inhibitor-I. This syndrome is now referred to as the Metabolic Syndrome or Insulin Resistance Syndrome.

Very Low Calorie Diet: A weight loss diet that provides fewer than 800 kcalories per day.

Weight Cycling or Yo-Yo Dieting: The repeated cycles of weight loss and regain, referred to as weight cycling or yo-yo dieting.

Appendix 4
Tips and Suggestions

1. A diet in a weight loss programme should meet all the nutrients except calories.
2. The diet plan should not be rigid.
3. A realistic goal for the weight loss should be set.
4. Increased physical activity should be the integral part of the weight loss programme.
5. A bowl of salads and a glass of water before lunch and dinner helps to cut down the food intake.
6. Include variety in the diet.
7. Avoid simultaneous actions, especially eating and watching TV.
8. Isolate the food so that the person needs to get up and collect the food.
9. Instead of using a difficult day as an excuse for overeating substitute other pleasures for reward.
10. Form a plan of action which helps you to respond to an environment where overeating is likely to happen especially in parties.
11. Include skimmed milk instead of whole milk.
12. Monitor the body weight at regular intervals and the diet be modified in case of increase in the weight.
13. Over and above "have patience". People often think of weight loss as a race, when actually it is a life long process.
14. Healthy eating does not mean to bid farewell to all the favourite foods. Nothing tasty has to be completely removed from eating plan, although high fat foods such as fast food and French fries must be kept to a minimum.
15. The initial goal of weight loss therapy should be to reduce body weight by about 10 percent from baseline.

16. Fat matters, but calories count.
17. Reducing dietary fat alone without reducing calories is not sufficient for weight loss. However, reducing dietary fat, along with reducing dietary carbohydrates, can help reduce calories.
18. The combination of a reduced calorie diet and increased physical activity is recommended since it produces weight loss that may also result in decrease in abdominal fat and increase in cardiorespiratory fitness.
19. Behaviour therapy is a useful adjunct when incorporated into treatment for weight loss and weight maintenance. Behaviour modification is easy to achieve when meditation is practised.
20. Eating healthy starts with healthy food shopping.

References

Journals

1. Aizawa – Abe M et. al., Pathophysiological Role of Leptin in Obesity Related Hypertension; *J Clin Invest,* 2000, 105(9), 1243-52.
2. Allison DB, KR Fontaine, JE Manson, J Stevens, TB VanItallie, Annual Deaths Attributable to Obesity in the United States, *JAMA,* 1999, 282(16), 1530-8.
3. Carin D, Childhood and Adolescent Obesity, *The Paediatric Clinics 15 (3),* August 2001, pp 227-233.
4. Charlotte MW, P Louise, L Douglas, WC Alan, 2002, Implications of Childhood.
5. Cicuttini FM, JR Baker, TD Spector, The Association of Obesity with Osteoarthritis of the Hand and Knee in Women – A Twin Study, *J Rheumatol,* 1996 23(7), 1221-6.
6. Deslypere JP, Obesity and Cancer, *Metabolism, 1995*; 44(9 *Suppl* 3): 24-27.
7. Fitzgibbon ML, MR Stolley, DS Kirschenhaum, An Obesity Prevention Pilot Programme in African-American Mothers and Daughters, *J Nutr Educ,* 1995, 27, 93-97.
8. Flier SF et. al., Obesity, *Harrison's Principle of Internal Medicine, 15 th edition,* 77: 479-486.
9. Foster JL, RW Jeffery, TL Schwd, FM Kramer, Preventing Weight Gain in Adults, A Pound of Prevention, *Health Psychology,* 1988, 7515-25.
10. G Ma, Y Li, Comparison of Overweight Prevalence by Different Standards in Chinese Adolescents, *Abstract in Proceedings of IX Asian Congress of Nutrition,* New Delhi, 2003, p 315.
11. G Ma, Y Li, Obesity Prevalence of Chinese Children Living in 4 Cities of China, *Abstract in Proceedings of IX Asian Congress of Nutrition,* New Delhi, 2003, p 315.

12. Garrow JS, Treatment of Obesity, Lancet, 1992, 340:409.
13. Ghani AN, AL Hee, Prevalence of Overweight and Its Associated Factors Amongst Urban Prepubertal Children in Malacca, Malaysia, *Abstract in Proceedings of IX Asian Congress of Nutrition*, New Delhi, p 328.
14. Gillis LJ, LC Kennedy, AM Gillis, Relationship Between Juvenile Obesity, Dietary Energy and Fat Intake and Physical Activity, *Int J Obes Relat Metab Disord*, 2002, 26(4); 458-63.
15. Giovannucci E et. al., Physical Activity, Obesity, and Risk for Colon Cancer and Adenoma in Men. *Ann Intern Med 1995*, 122(5):327-34.
16. Hessan MA, Obesity: An Emerging Health Problem In Asia, *Abstract in Proceedings of IX Asian Congress of Nutrition*, New Delhi, 2003, p 318.
17. Huang Z, SE Hankinson, GA Colditz, et. al. Dual Effects of Weight and Weight Gain on Breast Cancer Risk. *Journal of the American Medical Association*. 1997; 278:1407-1411.
18. Ismail MN, Obesity: An Emerging Public Health Problem in Asia, *Abstract, Symposium at IX Asian Congress of Nutrition*, New Delhi, 2003, p 70.
19. Jain S, B Pant, Adolescent Obesity in the Public Schools of Meerut, *Abstract in Proceedings of IX Asian Congress of Nutrition*, New Delhi, 2003, p 319.
20. Jeffery RW, SA French, Preventing Weight Gain in Adults, A Pound of Prevention, *Health Psychology*, 1999, 89, pp 747-51.
21. Kagdi H, RV Dosi, Clinical and Investigative Profile of Obese Patients, Department of Medicine, Medical College, Baroda, 2004.
22. Kamboj AK, et. al., Obesity in Meerut and Urban Perspective, *Abstract in Proceedings of IX Asian Congress of Nutrition*, New Delhi, 2003, p 321.
23. Kapur P, M Sethi, Dietary Profile and Physical Activity Pattern of Indian Obese Versus Normal Weight Children, *Abstract in Proceedings of IX Asian Congress of Nutrition*, New Delhi, 2003, p 322.
24. Kaur J, A Pandher, I Singh, Study of Childhood Obesity and Its Management, *Abstract in Proceedings of IX Asian Congress of Nutrition*, New Delhi, 2003, p 316.
25. Kim JH, SH Kim, CE Chung, CH Yu, JS Lee, Effects of Dietary Intakes, Food Behaviour and Lifestyle of Obesity of Korean Elementary Students, *Abstract in Proceedings of IX Asian Congress of Nutrition*, New Delhi, pp 326-27.

26. Kumari V, N Khurana, Abdominal Obesity Management by Transion N Europe Along With Dietary Advice and Guidance Among Urban Indians, *Abstract in Proceedings of IX Asian Congress of Nutrition*, New Delhi, 2003, p317.
27. Lee CD, SN Blair, AS Jackson, Cardiorespiratory Fitness, Body Composition and All Cause Cardiovascular Disease Mortality in Men, *Am J Clin Nutr 1999*, 69(3), 373-80.
28. Mabel D, Health Promotion Strategies to Reduce Obesity in Singapore, *Abstract, Symposium at IX Asian Congress of Nutrition*, New Delhi, 2003, p 70.
29. Manson JE et. al., Body Weight and Mortality Among Women, *N Engl J Med*, 1995, 333(11): 677-85.
30. Matkovic V et. al., Leptin is Inversely Related to Age at Menarche in Human Females, *J Clin Endorinol Metab 1997*, 82(10), 3239-45.
31. Micheal RO, L Rudolp, HI Jules, Obesity, *N Engl J Med., 1997*, 362:396-408.
32. Mirmiran P, F Mohammadi, N Sarbazi, F Azizi, Association of Overweight and Central Obesity With Other Cardiovascular Disease Risk Factors: Tehran Lipid and Glucose Study, *Abstract in Proceedings of IX Asian Congress of Nutrition*, New Delhi, pp 311-12.
33. Monga S, K Khanna, Obesity Among School Children (7-9 years) In Delhi: Prevalence and Related Factors, *Abstract in Proceedings of IX Asian Congress of Nutrition*, New Delhi, p 320.
34. Montague CT et. al., Congenital Leptin Deficiency is Associated with Severe Early Onset Obesity in Humans, *Nature, 1997*, 387(6636); 903-8.
35. Parimala R, P Vijayalakshme, BA Vasumathy, Allopathy Versus Naturopathy in the Treatment of Obesity and Developing: An Educational Package, *Abstract in Proceedings of IX Asian Congress of Nutrition*, New Delhi, 2003, p 317.
36. Patil JS, Naik RK, Prevalence and Assessment of Obesity Among Urban High School Children, *Abstract in Proceedings of IX Asian Congress of Nutrition*, New Delhi, 2003, p 318.
37. Peter B, K Denise, B Iain, Prevalence of Overweight and Obese Children between 1989 and 1998: Population Based Series of Cross-sectional Studies, *Selections from BMJ*, 17, 2001, pp 223 – 225.
38. Policy Statement, Identifying and Treating Eating Disorders, *Paediatrics*, 15 (3), 2003, pp 227-233.
39. Popkin BM, S Paeratakul, F Zhai, K Ge, Dietary and Environmental Correlates of Obesity in a Population Study in China, *Obes Res*, 1995, Suppl 2: 135-143.

40. Prabhjot S, Prevalance of Obesity Among the School Children of Amritsar City in Punjab, *Abstract in Proceedings of IX Asian Congress of Nutrition*, New Delhi, 2003, p 322.
41. Rahman SMM, Childhood Obesity in Dhaka City: Is It An Emerging Problem?, *Abstract in Proceedings of IX Asian Congress of Nutrition*, New Delhi, 2003, p 315.
42. Rahman SMM, et. al., Childhood Obesity In Dhaka City: Is It An Emerging Problem? 2003.
43. Reddy L, JM Begum, Abdominal Obesity Among Coronary Artery By-Pass Graft (CABG) Patients, *Abstract in Proceedings of IX Asian Congress of Nutrition*, New Delhi, p 320.
44. Richard AD et. al., AACE/ACE Position Statement on the Prevention, Diagnosis and Treatment of Obesity, 1998.
45. Saad MF et. al., Diurnal and Ultradian Rhythmicity of Plasma Leptin, Effects of Gender and Adiposity, *J Clin Endocrinol Metab 1998*, 83(2); 453-9.
46. Schoeller DA; LK Cella, MK Sinha, JF Caro, Entertainment of the Diurnal Rhythm of Plasma Leptin to Meal Timing, *J Clin Invest 1997*, 100(7), 1882-7.
47. Schwartz MB, R Puhl, Childhood Obesity: a Societal Problem to Solve, *Obesity Research 2003*: 4:57-71.
48. Sharma A, K Sharma, K Prasad, Obesity In Affluent Children, In Adolescents In Delhi, *Abstract in Proceedings of IX Asian Congress of Nutrition*, New Delhi, 2003, p. 318.
49. Sharma M, M Singh, Childhood Obesity and Contributory Factors, *Abstract in Proceedings of IX Asian Congress of Nutrition*, New Delhi, 2003, p 317.
50. Sheth M, Kaur J, Effectiveness of A Weight Reducing Clinic at Baroda, India, *Abstract in Proceedings of IX Asian Congress of Nutrition*, New Delhi, p 321.
51. Shetty P, Obesity in the Asian Region: Causes and Consequences, *Abstract, Symposium at IX Asian Congress of Nutrition*, New Delhi, 2003, p 69.
52. Sobal J, AJ Stunkard, Socioeconomic Status and Obesity, a Review of the Literature, *Psychol Bull*, 1989, 105: 260-275.
53. Sriram U, Childhood Obesity, *Indian Journal of Clinical Practice*, 12 (3), 2001, p 61-63.
54. Stampfer MJ; KM Maclure; GA Colditz; JE Manson; WC Willett; Risk of Symptomatic Gallstones in Women with Severe Obesity, *Am J Clin Nutr, 1992*; 55(3): 652-8.

55. Stevens J et. al., The Effect of Age on the Association Between Body Mass Index and Mortality, *N Engl J Med 1998*, 338(1), 1-7.
56. Stolley MR, ML Fitzzibbin, Effects of an Obesity Prevention Programme on the Eating Behaviour of African-American Mothers and their Daughters – *Health Educ Behav,* 24, 1997, pp 152-64.
57. Sundquist J, MA Winkleby, S Pudaric, Cardiovascular Disease Risk Factor Amongst Older Black, Mexican-American and White Women and Men, An Analysis of NHANES III, 1988-94, Third National Health and Nutrition Examination Survey, *J. Am, Geriatr. Soc,* 49:109-116, 2001.
58. Tessa JP, P Chris, M Orly, Fetal and Early Life Growth and Body Mass Index from Birth to Early Adulthood in 1958, British Cohort: Longitudinal Study, *Selections from BMJ,* 18, pp 38-42.
59. Trayhurn P, The Biology of Obesity—Recent Development in the Regulation of Energy Balance, *Abstract, Symposium at IX Asian Congress of Nutrition,* New Delhi, 2003, p 70.
60. Van der Kooy K, JC Seidell, Techniques for the Measurement of Visceral Fat; a Practical Guide, *Int J Obes Relat Metab Disord* 1993, 17(4), 187-96.
61. Vedavati S, R Jayashree, R Mohammad, Prevalence of Overweight and Obesity in Affluent Adolescent Girls in Chennai in 1981 and 1998, *Indian Paediatrics,* 40, 2003, pp 332-336.
62. Wei M et. al., Relationship between Low Cardiore-spiratory Fitness and Mortality in Normal Weight, Overweight and Obese Men, *JAMA 1999,* 282(16), 1547-53.
63. Weigle DS; PB Duell; WE Connor; RA Steiner; MR Soules; JL Kuijper: Effect of Fasting, Refeeding and Dietary Fat Restriction on Plasma Leptin Levels. *J Clin Endocrinol Metab* 1997, 82(2): 561-5.
64. Wilson DC, Obesity in Childhood – Much More Than A Cosmetic Problem, *J R Coll Physicians Edinb,* 36, 2004, pp 6-10.
65. Wilson GT, CA Nonas, GD Rosenblum, Assessment of Binge eating in Obese Patients, *Int J Eat Disord,* 1993, 13-25-33.
66. Yoshiike N, Increasing Obesity in Men and Undernutrition in Women – A Japanese Paradox, *Abstract, Symposium at IX Asian Congress of Nutrition,* New Delhi, 2003, p 71.
67. Zohourian G, Navai L, Prevalence of Obesity and Hypertension In Patients With Type 2 Diabetes, *Abstract in Proceedings of IX Asian Congress of Nutrition,* New Delhi, p 312.
68. ZX Yang, Relationship Between Obesity and Correlative Chronic Diseases in Chinese Adults, *Abstract in Proceedings of IX Asian Congress of Nutrition,* New Delhi, 2003, p 315.

Books Referred

I. Brown JE, *Nutrition Now*, An International Thomson Publishing Company, 1998.

II. Desai BB, *Handbook of Nutrition and Diet*, Marcel Dekker, Inc., New York, 2000.

III. Garrow JS, *Obesity, Human Nutrition and Dietitics*, 9th edition, (JS Garrow)

IV. Indian Council Of Medical Research, *Nutrient Requirements And Recommended Dietary Allowances For Indians*, National Institute of Nutrition, Hyderabad, 2002.

V. Martorell R, International Food Policy Research Institute, 2001.

VI. National Institute of Nutrition, *Dietary Guidelines for Indians, A Manual*, NIN, Hyderabad, 1999.

VII. Oser Bernard L, *Hawk's Physiological Chemistry*, Tata Mc Graw Hill Publishing Company Ltd., Bombay, 1965.

VIII. Park K, *Parks Textbook Of Preventive And Social Medicine*, Banarsidas Bhanot Publishers, Jabalpur, 1995.

IX. Rohinson Corinne H, Marilyn R. Lawler, Normal and Therapeutic Nutrition, Oxford & IBH Publishing Co., New Delhi, 1982.

X. Smolin LA, MB Grossvenor, *Nutrition Science And Applications*, Saunders College Publishing, Harcourt Brace College Publishers, 1997.

XI. Srilakshmi, B, *Dietetics*, New Age International (P) Ltd., Publishers, New Delhi, 2000.

XII. Srilaxhmi B, *Nutrition Science*, New Age International (P) Limited, Publishers, New Delhi, 2002.

XIII. Swaminathan M, *Essentials of Food and Nutrition, Volume I & II*. The Bangalore Printing and Publishing Co. Ltd., Bangalore, 1988.

XIV. Williams Sue Rodwell, *Nutrition & Diet Therapy*, Timer Mirror / Mosby College Publishing St. Louis, 1985.

XV. WPT James ed. *Churchill Livingstone*, Edinburgh, London, 1993, p 465.

Internet

(i) http://www.niddk.nih.gov/health/nutrit/pubs/unders.htm
(ii) http://www.weight.com/definition.asp
(iii) NIDDK Weight-Control Information Network
(iv) http://www.medivisionindia.com/nutrition/obesity.phtml
(v) http://pib.nic.in/release/release.asp?relid=1048
(vi) http://health.indiatimes.com/articleshow/407600.cms
(vii) http://www.indiainfoline.com/nevi/lamm.html
(viii) http://www.niddk.nih.gov/health/nutrit/pubs/unders.htm
(ix) http://www.weight.com/definition.asp
(x) www.about-obesity.com
(xi) http://www.bnaiyer.com/health
(xii) http://www.mirror-mirror.org/men.htm
(xiii) http://www.eating-disorders.com/Obsessing.cfm
(xiv) http://www.nedic.ca/glossary.html
(xv) http://www.nlm.nih.gov/medlineplus/eatingdisorders.html
(xvi) http://www.nimh.nih.gov/publicat/eatingdisorders.cfm
(xvii) http://www.mentalhealth.org/publications/allpubs/ken98-0047/default.asp
(xviii) http://www.kjwebproductions.com
(xix) http:// www.disability.vic.gov.au/dsonline/dsarticles.nsf/pages/Hormones_obesity? Open Document
(xx) http://www.who.int/archives/inf-pr-1997/en/pr97-46.html
(xxi) http://advance.uri.edu/pacer/june2002/story12.htm
(xxii) http://diabetes.niddk.nih.gov/dm/pubs/statistics/index.htm.
(xxiii) www.fao.org/FOCUS/E/obesity/obes1.htm
(xxiv) Wellness International Network Ltd - web.winltd.com